Understanding
CHRONIC
PAIN

Understanding
CHRONIC
PAIN

A Doctor Talks
To His Patients

ROBERT T. COCHRAN JR., M.D.

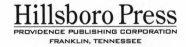
Hillsboro Press
PROVIDENCE PUBLISHING CORPORATION
FRANKLIN, TENNESSEE

Printed in the United States of America

08   07   06   05   04   1   2   3   4   5

Library of Congress Catalog Card Number: 2003112449

ISBN: 1-57736-302-7

Cover design by Kelly Bainbridge

HILLSBOROPRESS
an imprint of
Providence Publishing Corporation
238 Seaboard Lane • Franklin, Tennessee 37067
www.providence-publishing.com
800-321-5692

To those who suffer chronic pain
and do not understand why.

Contents

Acknowledgments

This is a book about chronic pain, written largely by those who suffer the disease. I have merely transcribed their stories, altering them only to disguise identities. The stories are true and the people are real. My debt to them for what they have taught me is incalculable.

I am indebted also to those colleagues who have referred to me the most difficult clinical problems imaginable. We have attempted together to fathom the mystery of chronic pain. One of the delights of my professional life has been to watch them grow in understanding, as I myself have grown.

My wife, Donna, has given me time and space as I have pursued the fundamentally selfish act of writing this book. My appreciation for that simple act of courtesy is very great indeed. Two of my children, Heather and Chuck, are published authors and they have been instrumental in seeing this work to press. Andrew Miller and the staff at Providence Publishing Corporation have been very helpful. Sherry Jolly, my transcriptionist, has been of invaluable assistance, not only in her professional skills, but in her unfailing good humor. Janet Epstein has proofed this book through many revisions, and without her it simply could not have been written. Kristie Renardson, Jan Diehl, Linda Harris, Pat Lovell, and Jennifer Hargrove have helped me care for many victims of chronic pain. They have taught me that in the treatment of the painful, nothing is quite as important as patience.

This manuscript has been reviewed by physicians and lay-persons alike. In order to spare them any personal embarrassment

Understanding Chronic Pain

or responsibility for ideas that may be uniquely my own, I will keep them nameless. They know who they are and they know of my gratitude. I will prepare the reader for that which follows by noting that some reviewers have greeted this work with enthusiasm and others have expressed offense at my judgments. I accept both opinions with equal appreciation, secure in the knowledge that a book about a subject as controversial as chronic pain cannot satisfy everyone.

My last acknowledgment, and a fitting introduction to this book, is to Dr. John Shapiro. I came under his tutelage nearly fifty years ago as a student at the Vanderbilt University School of Medicine. He was the greatest of my teachers, and he gave me the single most valuable lesson I would ever learn as a physician. He demanded that *I must record what I see, not what I am supposed to see.* That dictum has served me well, and I have obeyed it in writing this book. I write about what I see chronic pain to be, not what others see it to be. For this reason I make no reference to the work of authorities in the field, nor do I offer a bibliography.

Drugs Useful for Pain

M ost of the drugs discussed in this book are identified by their trademarked, proprietary names. A few, those whose usage extends over several decades, are identified by their generic. I have chosen that form that I find most recognizable by patients and physicians. I have placed those drug names of universal recognition, such as morphine and alcohol, in the lower case and all others in capitals. This avoids the thought-interrupting alteration of the upper case for proprietary and lower case for generic drugs.

	PROPRIETARY	GENERIC
Opiate Analgesics	Demerol	Meperidine
	Dilaudid	Hydromorphone
	Duragesic	Fentanyl
	Lortab, Vicodin	Hydrocodone
	MS Contin, Kadian	Morphine
	Percodan, Tylox, Oxycontin	Oxycodone
Opiate-like Analgesics	Darvon	Propoxyphene
	Nubain	Nalbuphine
	Stadol	Butorphanol
	Ultram	Tramadol
Tricyclic Antidepressants	Anafranil	Clomipramine
	Elavil	Amitriptyline
	Pamelor	Nortriptyline
	Sinequan	Doxepin
	Tofranil	Imipramine

	PROPRIETARY	GENERIC
Selective Serotonin Reuptake Inhibitors (Antidepressant)	Celexa Luvox Paxil Prozac Zoloft	Citalopram Fluvoxamine Paroxetine Fluoxetine Sertraline
Benzodiazepines (Anxiolytic and Anticonvulsant)	Ativan Klonopin Valium Xanax	Lorazepam Clonazepam Diazepam Alprazolam
Anticonvulsants (also Antimanic and Antimigraine)	Depakote Dilantin Lamictal Neurontin Tegretol Topamax	Valproate Phenytoin Lamotrigine Gabapentin Carbamazepine Topiramate
Membrane Stabilizers (Antimanic and Antimigraine)	Lithonate, Eskalith	Lithium
Phenothiazines (Antipsychotics)	Stelazine Trilafon Thorazine Triavil (Combination)	Trifluoperazine Perphenazine Chlorpromazine Perphenazine and Amitriptyline
Atypical Antipsychotics (also Antimanic)	Risperdal Seroquel Zyprexa	Risperidone Quetiapine Olanzapine
Stimulants	Adderall Dexedrine Ritalin	Amphetamine Dextroamphetamine Methylphenidate

Introduction

I am a physician, trained in internal medicine. My competence extends also to the fields of neurology, psychiatry, and neuropharmacology. I began those studies years ago when my endeavor to understand the nature of chronic pain began in earnest.

From time immemorial, pain has been recognized as the cardinal sign of injury to the body. This is not always so. Some people experience pain, often for a lifetime, after complete recovery from injury, and others with disorders such as fibromyalgia and tension headache suffer pain in the absence of any identifiable injury. This state of unaccountable pain has long defied explanation. Only within the past couple of decades have we come to recognize it as a unique illness, with its own natural history and pattern of clinical behavior.

The study of chronic pain is a new and rapidly expanding medical discipline. The emergence of molecular biology has offered remarkable insights into the biochemical reactions which occur within the brain and the body in those experiencing pain. Much has been learned and more will be. Nonetheless, we must recognize that at this time medical science knows less about chronic pain than it does about cancer, heart disease, or any other major illness. As every physician knows, the care of the painful patient can be a frustrating and humbling pursuit.

This is a personal narrative, a record of my passage among victims of chronic pain and the discoveries that have come from those encounters. I write for physicians, nurses, therapists, and caregivers, but mostly I write for you who suffer the disease. I know you very well, perhaps as well as anybody in the world. I have listened to your stories with patience and attention, and I have been greatly rewarded. You have trusted me and invited me to share the dark recesses of your thoughts and fears and the memories of the dreadful experiences that are so often the origin of chronic pain. I have treated thousands of you and I believe that I have some understanding of your illness. I certainly understand the sense of self-doubt and indignity that comes with it. I have heard you say many times, "I am a *strong* person. Why has this happened to me?"

I describe many diseases. Some—fibromyalgia and headache—are common. Others, less so, are known only to those who suffer the strange and exotic illness. I illustrate some of the unusual and bizarre examples of chronic pain, for the uncommon clinical event often helps us understand the common. I explore the role of pharmacy in the treatment of pain and the role of destructive life events in its genesis. My book is a series of essays, not about painful diseases, but about painful patients. From the study of their case histories I derive certain conclusions. Some are bold. Some are frightful. Some may be amusing. Some are certainly wrong, but I believe most are right.

While it is inherently attractive to treat illness by lifestyle modification and the power of the spirit, we need to be reminded that there are few diseased that in this era cannot be treated rather well by pharmacy.

Be advised that this is not a book for the faint-hearted. It is a serious study of science, intended for serious people. I will ask quite a lot of you for, of necessity, I must explore the arcane worlds of neuroscience and neuropharmacology. I will do this unobtrusively and carefully, confident that you will be able to follow the development of my ideas. I know that you are informed and knowledgeable, and that you will not be intimidated by medical jargon. You already know many of the terms. You talk the talk. I make reference to the drugs used in the treatment of pain, and for your convenience they are listed in this preface. You will not be unnecessarily challenged by their names. Certainly, you have taken many of them.

I have learned many important lessons as a practicing physician. One of the greatest of these is that I must never underestimate the intelligence of my patient. I do not intend to underestimate the intelligence of my reader. I do not suggest that this book offers the easy answer or the quick cure to chronic pain. It is beneath my dignity, and yours, to do so. Chronic pain, as you certainly know, is a vastly complex illness. Indeed, *it is the most complex of all diseases*. It has many origins and many behaviors, and it responds, as does no other disease, to drugs of incredible variety.

The use of drugs in the treatment of pain has received little attention in the popular press. Most books on the subject embrace non-pharmacologic therapies such as dietary modification, exercise, physical therapy, and the employ of spiritual awakening and empowerment. These can certainly be of benefit in the treatment of pain, but they can be of equal benefit in the treatment of almost any disease. There is no need, I suggest, to single out chronic pain as a disorder that is uniquely responsive to non-pharmacologic therapy. While it is inherently attractive to treat illness by lifestyle modification and the power of the spirit, we need to be reminded that there are few diseased that in this era cannot be treated rather well by pharmacy. Who, in their right mind, would suggest that we discard drug therapy in the treatment of diabetes, arthritis, or heart failure? Who would suggest, and here we move closer to the mark, that we discard pharmacy in the treatment of depression? Or schizophrenia, epilepsy, or manic-depressive illness? This is not to denigrate the value of non-pharmacologic treatments. They can be very helpful, but as many readers know, they are often not adequate for the relief of pain. Therefore we must, of necessity, rely on drugs, and what's so bad about that? We rely on them for the treatment of most diseases.

I acknowledge that the utility of drugs in the treatment of pain is limited. Even in the best of hands, they really work only about half of the time. This pales next to the success rate that can be achieved with the use of drugs for diabetes, arthritis, and heart failure. Should a success rate of only 50 percent dissuade us from their use? It would if there were better treatments, but there are not. The success rate of non-pharmacologic therapies is certainly no greater than 50 percent and probably much less than that. The role of pharmacy in the treatment of chronic pain is a central theme of this book. There are many drugs that offer enormous promise, not just in relieving pain but in helping us to *understand the fundamental nature of the disease.*

In the course of this work, I will compare pain, its origins, its natural history, and its response to treatment to those of other diseases. To begin, I will go back in time to nearly half a century ago, the point at which this book really begins. Two of the most destructive illnesses with which physicians contended then (and still do) were schizophrenia and depression. They were mysterious and unfathomable disorders. There was absolutely no understanding of the biochemical reactions that dictated their strange behaviors. Then there came, largely by accident, the discovery of drugs which at least partially ameliorated their malevolence. They weren't perfect drugs (even now no drug is perfect) and their performance was spotty. They only worked about half the time, but they created a revolution and a new science, that which we know as neuropharmacology. As the understanding of the biochemical actions of the drugs evolved, so did the understanding of schizophrenia and depression. As so often happens in clinical medicine, it was the chance discovery of a drug that led to the understanding of the fundamental nature of a disease. Where we stood fifty years ago with depression and schizophrenia is about where we stand today with chronic pain—but not quite. Back then we had only one or two drugs for each disorder. Today we have many drugs, of great variety, useful in the treatment of chronic pain. Most of them, as you probably know, began their careers in the treatment of other diseases, several of them mental.

Bruce had a youthful, handsome face. There was an air of confidence and ability about him, and he moved with fluidity and grace, unusual for a painful patient. I suspected that he was an athlete, a golfer perhaps.

"How long have you had pain?"

"Most of my life. I played football in college and had a couple of knee operations. My knees still hurt, but most of my pain has been in my back. I'm sure it is due to the G-forces. I have spent a lot time at 6 or 7 Gs."

"G-forces?"

"Yeah, I was a Marine pilot. I flew the F-16. That plane is rough on the body. Whenever I got to high Gs my back would really hurt."

"How long were you in the Marines?"

"Twenty years. I spent the last five as an instructor before I had to retire."

"Did you retire because of your pain?"

"No, I'd never let a little pain keep me from flying. It was something else. About two years ago I was instructing a student, and I suddenly fell asleep in the cockpit. The doctors worked me up and told me that I had sleep apnea. They said I had a blockage in my throat and that kept me from sleeping well at night. That's why I was sleepy during the day. They operated on me to open up the back of my throat so I could breathe better when I slept."

"Did that help?"

"Yeah, it did help some, but not near as much as they told me it would. I still get sleepy from time to time. If I had a choice again, I wouldn't have accepted the operation. I would have had to retire anyway."

"And then?"

"I became a stockbroker and a developer."

"You did both?"

"Yeah, I have always had lots of energy. I enjoy being busy."

"Property development is pretty risky business. Why did you get into that?"

"Doc, my middle name is risk. Besides, it didn't take much money. I bought some land, rented a bulldozer, and started clearing it."

"By yourself?"

"Yeah, I wanted to build an apartment house."

"Bruce, let me get this straight. You were a combat fighter pilot. You developed sleep apnea and had to leave the service. You began a new career as a stockbroker and at the same time started building an apartment house in your spare time. Is that correct?"

"Yeah, that's right. I hated to leave the service, but I was excited about my new life."

"Let's get back to the pain, Bruce. Tell me how it began."

"My back bothered me for years. Most of the time it wasn't too bad. Like I told you, it only really hurt when I flew, but by the time I retired it was hurting all the time. I figured that my back would get better when I stopped flying, but it didn't. I gave up bulldozing, but that didn't help either. The pain kept getting worse, and it started shooting down into my left leg. One day the leg went numb and my foot was paralyzed. An MRI showed a ruptured disc, and I had surgery the next day."

"Did the operation help you?"

"Yeah, the feeling in my leg and the strength came back real good, but my back pain continued. It even spread into my shoulder blades and sometimes into my neck. When that happened I would get a headache. The pain even went into my hands. They got numb and tingly."

"On both sides?"

"Yeah, both sides."

"What happened then?"

"Let me tell him, honey," said his wife. "He started drinking. He drank way too much."

"Had that been a problem before?"

"Not really. He would go on binges from time to time. He didn't get drunk very often, but when he did he did a pretty good job of it. After the operation, he drank beer all the time. He said his pain was unbearable, and the only way he could relieve it was by drinking. He couldn't play with the children any more. Many times I would see him sitting alone in a dark room, crying. He was very depressed."

"And then?"

"It was on Memorial Day, just about six months ago. Bruce told me that he was going to commit suicide."

"What did you do?"

"I called our internist."

"I love that man," interjected Bruce. "He saved my life, at least what's left of it. He is my hero."

"What did the internist do?"

The wife took over. "He sent us to the emergency room and arranged for a psychiatric consultation. Bruce was admitted to the hospital. He was there for a week. The psychiatrist told us that Bruce had manic-depressive illness. He prescribed Depakote and Risperdal."

"Did the drugs help?"

"Yes, they helped a lot. There was no more talk of suicide, and Bruce was able to stop drinking. The drugs seemed to even him out. He used to be very moody, sometimes up, sometimes down. He is not that way anymore."

"And the pain?"

"It's still there, and worse than ever. Sometimes it actually feels like I have a hot poker in my back. I don't have any appetite and I am really fatigued. I don't even want sex anymore. I am too tired. The pain has really beaten me down."

"I'll guess you are having trouble sleeping."

"I sleep fair now, but for a while I couldn't sleep at all. The psychiatrist gave me Trazodone, but that didn't help."

"You said you are sleeping better now. How did that come about?"

"It was the Klonopin. As soon as I got on Klonopin I started sleeping better."

"The psychiatrist gave you Klonopin?"

"No, it was the otologist."

"The otologist! How did an otologist get involved?"

"Because of the tinnitus. I had this terrible sound in my ears. It was a constant buzzing. It began a few weeks before I went into the psych unit, and it was driving me crazy. I think it was because of that as much as the pain that I wanted to commit suicide. The otologist told me I had inflammation in my inner ear and treated me with Klonopin. That was about three months ago. The tinnitus went away, and I was able to sleep a little bit better. That otologist is a real hero."

"That is quite a story, Bruce. You certainly had an interesting year."

"Yeah," he grimaced, "quite a year."

"What are you taking for your pain?"

"My internist gave me Percodan, and it helps some, but I don't want to take it. I realize that I was addicted to alcohol, and I am afraid of becoming addicted to Percodan."

"It was your neurosurgeon who sent you to me. What was his take on your pain?"

"I have been seeing him all along since the operation. Every time I went to him, I hoped he would find something he could operate on, but he told me that all my tests were normal, that my back was just fine. He couldn't explain the pain. He thought that maybe I had something called fibromyalgia. He did do some electrical tests on my hands and told me that they showed carpal tunnel syndrome. That was why my hands were burning. I asked him if he could fix it, and he said something that surprised me. He told me he could do the operation very easily, but that he couldn't guarantee the outcome. He said that he had relieved pressure on a nerve in my back, and I had not gotten better. He was afraid that I wouldn't get any better after he relieved pressure on the nerves in my wrists. He advised that I see a pain specialist before undertaking any more surgery."

The neurosurgeon, aware of the strange turns that Bruce's life had taken, and aware also that there is sometimes more to pain than pinched nerves was the real hero.

"Can you help me, Doc?"

"Yes, Bruce, almost certainly."

Had I seen Bruce a few years ago, I would not have been able to say that. I would have been lost in a forest of clinical details. It would have been quite impossible to make sense out of the incredible variety of his illnesses. He suffered lumbar disc disease, carpal tunnel syndrome, fibromyalgia, tinnitus, alcoholism, depression to the point of suicidal ruminations, and manic grandiosity in trying to build an apartment house in his spare time. I know now that Bruce didn't have lots of different diseases. He had a single core illness, chronic pain.

Not too long ago, my success rate in treating pain was about 25 percent. Today it is closer to 60 percent. I am armed with the knowledge that comes from experience, and I was able to offer Bruce the greatest gift a patient with chronic pain can ever receive, the hope of getting well. I prescribed the drug Imipramine and instructed him to take a small amount at first but to gradually increase the dosage, all the while continuing his other medicines. I also asked Bruce if he would be interested in reading a book about chronic pain, written by a doctor for his patients. He accepted my manuscript.

When Bruce and his wife returned two weeks later, he extended his hand and said, "I think I am getting better."

"Tell me about it."

"The pain doesn't bother me as much. It's going away from my neck and shoulders, and my hands don't tingle the way they used to. I have more energy. I even played with my kids a little bit. I haven't done that in nearly a year."

I know now that Bruce didn't have lots of different diseases. He had a single core illness, chronic pain.

"Are you sleeping better?"

"Yeah, a lot. My muscles used to jerk all through the night. That doesn't happen anymore. Now, when I wake up, I feel more rested. When can I get back to work?"

"Not yet, Bruce, but perhaps pretty soon. Let's not rush things. There are going to be some bumps in the road yet, but I am sure you will get well."

"Will I have to keep taking these medicines?"

"Yes, you will have to take your medicines probably for the rest of your life. It is a small price to pay. Go ahead and get used to it."

"I liked your book, Doc. It was Shack-Bull."

"What is Shack-Bull?"

"Sorry, that's pilot talk. It means hitting the target dead on."

"He devoured it," said his wife. "He made a lot of marginal notes and underlines."

"Yeah, I did. Fighter pilots are anal retentive."

"You read the piece about the insurance salesman with pain, manic-depressive disease, and tinnitus?"

"Yeah, I liked that. He was a lot like me, wasn't he?"

"Yes, almost exactly like you."

"And he got well, didn't he?"

"He certainly got a lot better. Now tell me, Bruce, were there parts of the book that you didn't like. Were there parts that bothered you?"

"Yeah, a lot of it bothered me. The chapter on childhood abuse really got to me. I had trouble reading it. I had to walk away several times."

"I can guess why. Do you mind telling me about it?"

"My parents loved me, Doc, and I still love them, but they were way too rough on me. I got whipped a lot. It still hurts—real bad—when I think about it. I would never treat my kids the way I was treated."

"Do you feel like you were abused?"

"Yeah, I hate to use the word, but yes, I was abused."

"How long did it go on?"

"Until I was ten years old. My mother was whipping me, and I grabbed the belt away and started whipping her. There were no more beatings after that."

It is people like Bruce about whom and for whom I write. I have interviewed and treated many of you, and I count that experience the most rewarding of my professional life. By sharing your stories and analyzing your response to drugs and, perhaps equally importantly, your lack of response to drugs, we can, I believe, reach some understanding of the true nature of chronic pain. As I present your case histories, I will offer my judgments. I ask you to read critically and reach your own.

You will, I'm sure, find yourself in the patients I describe in this book. The encounters may not be pleasant. Nonetheless, if you read with an open mind, free of prejudice and preconception, I think you will acquire some insights into an illness that really may not be what you think it is.

Understanding
CHRONIC
PAIN

CHAPTER ONE

Failure to Recover

T he body is able, at least over the short-term, to protect itself from pain. Most of us are aware that an acute injury can be quite painless. This effect is sometimes dramatic, particularly when the wound is severe. A youngster was involved in an automobile accident. An unrestrained passenger, he was thrown forward, his head into the windshield and his knee into the dash. He was concussed, lacerated, and fractured—his femur broken into two pieces. When we talked about the accident during his convalescence, he told me, "Dad, when I woke up on that pavement, I didn't hurt at all. I felt good. It was wonderful. I never had a feeling like that before."

The strange sense of well-being which may accompany major injury is mediated, as most of us know, by the release within the brain of chemicals known as endorphins. Metabolic energy is directed to the stabilization of injured tissue rather than being dissipated in pain, anxiety, and apprehension. It happens quickly and automatically. We cannot will it. It is nature's gift to us.

The analgesic and euphoric effect of the endorphins is duplicated by morphine. The drug deceives the body to its benefit by replicating nature's agency for the relief of pain. An attribute of the opioid effect, whether indigenous (endorphin) or exogenous (morphine) is that it is short-lived. It has to be. A state of analgesia and euphoria, so valuable in the face of overwhelming injury, cannot be sustained. Vigilance, attention, and awareness are lost, and that is detrimental. The being can no longer react appropriately to its environment.

Nature, with its fail-safe capacity for redundancy, has endowed us with a second system of analgesia. This employs the chemicals serotonin, noradrenaline, and probably several others. This system is operative over the long-term. Unlike the quick release, all or nothing opioid system, it is the day-in, day-out modulator of our awareness of pain. And, like the opioid system, it functions automatically.

The ability to tolerate pain is traditionally viewed in a psychologic or spiritual context. Strength of character, mind over matter, and all that. In truth, most of this occurs at a subconscious level. It is a biologic, not an emotional, attribute. It is our genetic heritage. We are empowered by our subconscious to dampen and modulate unnecessary sensation. We do not suffer severe and protracted pain every time we stub our toe any more than we enter a major depression with every emotional slight.

There are gradations in the severity of chronic pain, but in its fullest expression, it is a spirit-draining, soul-destroying illness.

The painful experience is usually brief, often just a few days. With severe injury such as a burn or fracture, it may persist for weeks or even months, but sooner or later it goes away. The wound heals, and pain dissipates. Indeed, pain is usually gone even before tissue recovery is complete. Sometimes, however, pain continues even after anatomic recovery. This is a common medical phenomenon. There are innumerable failure-to-recover syndromes, each with its own distinctive nomenclature. I will list a few and introduce the reader to the many varieties of chronic pain.

Shingles is an infection of peripheral nerves caused by the herpes zoster virus. It is characterized by a painful rash, and is a very distressing and destructive experience. Most people recover in a very few weeks. A minority, however, suffer ongoing pain even after the rash has disappeared, the disorder we know as post-herpetic neuralgia.

A bony fracture may evolve into a relentless syndrome of painfulness characterized by diminished blood flow, skin and muscular atrophy, contractures, and deformity, these occurring in spite of complete healing of the original injury. This dreadful disorder is recognized as reflex sympathetic dystrophy.

Lumbar disc disease is a common cause of back pain. In most cases it resolves with the passage of time, but if it does not, the herniated disc may be surgically removed. This usually meets with success but occasionally pain continues even though full anatomic repair has been achieved. This failure-to-recover syndrome is identified with the simple descriptor, the failed back.

Endometriosis is a painful affliction of women caused by the implantation of uterine tissue onto the pelvic floor. This tissue can be excised, but the disease often recurs, and multiple operations are necessary. Not infrequently, pain continues in spite of removal of all endometrial tissue. This is recognized, somewhat unimaginatively, as chronic pelvic pain. It might better be called the failed pelvis.

Migraine is a disease state characterized by episodic head pain, typically with intervals of well-being between attacks. In some patients the headache becomes transformed into an incessant painfulness without intervals of wellness. This disorder carries many names—tension headaches, chronic daily headache, or perhaps best, transformed migraine.

Muscular pain due to a sprain or overuse is extraordinarily common. The vast majority of patients recover with time and rest. In some, however, pain becomes chronic and incessant, the disorder that we call fibromyalgia.

There are countless other examples of chronic pain, but the point is made. A small subset of patients simply fail to recover from their painful experience, and chronic pain, in one of its many guises, ensues. This phenomenon, it bears emphasis, occurs indiscriminately. *Each and every painful experience carries with it the potential to persist in spite of anatomic recovery.*

There are gradations in the severity of chronic pain, but in its fullest expression, it is a spirit-draining, soul-destroying illness. Pain is incessant, and sleeplessness, fatigue, and despondency pervasive. The very fabric of a meaningful, integrated existence is unraveled. So alien to their experience is the state of painfulness that many patients wonder if they are not possessed of some form of madness. Not a few contemplate suicide.

Pain is a very depressing experience and chronic pain is, in the minds of many, an expression of depressive illness. This belief has been reinforced by the observation that certain drugs known as the tricyclic antidepressants are useful in the treatment of pain. These agents, introduced nearly fifty years ago, can often provide restoration of sleep, improvement in mood, and in some cases actual reduction of pain. The tricyclic drugs seem, for lack of a better word, to help the patient cope with pain. And there the matter rests. Some people fail to recover from painful disorders, become depressed, and can be helped—at least a bit—by antidepressant drug therapy. This, of course, doesn't really tell us why ongoing pain occurs. It only tells us how we behave when we become painful.

Acute pain is almost invariably the product of tissue injury. Whether due to a heart attack, kidney stone, or a muscle sprain, it has a recognizable cause. Remarkably, the cause of chronic pain is often not so clearly evident. This is the reason painful patients consume such an enormous share of medical resources. The search for the etiology of painfulness enlists many diagnostic procedures and its treatment many surgical operations. Sometimes the answer is found, but often not. In spite of the best efforts of the physician, chronic pain escapes precise definition and treatment.

I attend many patients with cancer, stroke, and heart disease. These people, who know they are likely to die of their illness, are accepting, unquestioning, and trustful. They understand the nature of their disease and their behavior, most of the time, is one of quiet dignity. Patients with chronic pain, who do not understand the nature of their illness, exhibit quite a different behavior. They will live, rather than die, with their fibromyalgia, chronic headaches, or back pain, and they are unsettled, questioning, suspicious, and often angry. Their pain is so intrusive and commanding and so often inexplicable that they obsess about it. They are frequently compulsive diarists and record keepers. Pain, more than any other chronic illness, produces a sort of mind warp in its victims. In their mental constructions, they present the physician not with their symptoms, but rather their conclusions. "No, I don't sleep, but it is just because the pain keeps me awake." "Sure, I have gained weight, but it's because I can't do anything. It hurts too much." "Yes, I am tired all the time, but you would be too if you hurt like I do." The anger can be palpable, and it finds direction toward those who they feel are responsible for their condition, the driver of the other car, the employer who terminated them, the insurance company that denied them their just benefits, or the doctor who won't or can't cure them. "Why that man even told me it was in my head. I am not crazy. I just hurt. This pain is real! Don't you understand?" The grimacing and wincing and protective postures, known as pain behaviors, imply exaggeration, and the demand for relief often becomes highly personal. "Doctor, you have got to give me something to relieve my pain." An unhappy interface, a painful patient, and an impotent physician.

Forty years ago, when I became a doctor, we didn't recognize that painfulness was an illness. Those who suffered with chronic pain were just an assembly of unfortunates who failed to respond to conventional treatments. We hadn't put it all together. We had not recognized that patients with fibromyalgia, headaches, or any of the many other disorders of chronic pain all exhibited very similar and predictable clinical behaviors, and that these behaviors, as complex and sometimes as unpleasant as they might be, merited study for what they were, the symptoms of a disease.

Physicians are now beginning to understand that chronic pain is an important—and common—disorder. The failed back is no longer a back problem. It is a pain problem. Chronic headache is no longer migraine. It is a pain problem, and the same for fibromyalgia and all the rest. We are beginning, only just beginning, to study painful behavior as a symptom of a disease and to realize that when the experience of pain persists beyond accountability, when the patient fails to recover, something profound is happening.

The syndrome of chronic pain is, as yet, a vague entity. It is a new disease, and our understanding is still evolving. One thing is certain, however—painful patients all exhibit similar behaviors. When acute pain becomes chronic, clinical behavior becomes very stereotyped.

Chronic pain rarely stays at the site of the original injury. It tends to move to adjacent body parts and with great frequency crosses the midline to involve, often quite symmetrically, the opposite side. Chronic pain confined to a single body part is quite rare. Often the entire body becomes painful.

Chronically painful patients are sleep-deprived in distinctive ways. There are frequent awakenings with painfulness, and pain often worsens at night. Sleep is interrupted by repetitive large muscle contractions called myoclonus, and attempts to sleep may be disturbed by a sense of having to constantly move the lower extremities, the restless legs phenomenon.

Painful patients are appetite-disordered. Weight loss may occur but more often weight gain. They can become very obese.

Painful patients experience, universally, fatigue and anergy (want of energy), and often changes in temperament and mood. Some become apathetic, others restless and hyperactive.

These are the identifiers of chronic pain. As diagnostic criteria, they may seem scant, but in their uniformity they are quite sufficient to accord the phenomenon of chronic pain the appellation of a disease entity.

CHAPTER TWO

What is Chronic Pain?

P ain is a universal human experience. We all know what it is like. Few of us, however, know enervating and debilitating chronic pain. What is it that distinguishes the disease chronic pain from the inevitable and sometimes incessant pain that we all endure? It is difficult to make a certain distinction. Unfortunately, there is as yet no adequate definition of the disease. The reasons for this are several, and they are worth exploring.

Chronic pain is a very protean illness. It has many faces. It may appear as fibromyalgia, back pain, tension headache, or any of the myriad other painful disorders. Thus, our attempt to define the illness is much like the proverbial blind men trying to describe the elephant. Each recognizes a part, none identify the whole. We can actually name the blind men. One is a rheumatologist who describes fibromyalgia. Another, an orthopedist, who describes a ruptured lumbar disc. A gynecologist describes chronic pelvic pain; a neurologist, tension headache; and a psychiatrist, depression. The list could be extended indefinitely. Every physician, specialist or generalist, encounters the syndrome of chronic pain. Each sees a piece of it. Few see the whole.

Let's compare chronic pain with cancer and infectious disease, for these, too, are very protean illnesses. There are many types of cancer, and they behave quite differently. There are many types of infectious disease. Some are caused by viruses, others by bacteria, and yet others by fungi. According to the type of organism, infections will show enormous variability in their clinical behaviors. Nonetheless, we recognize that cancer and infection each represent a single core disease. We know this because we can see, under the microscope, the nature of the illness. We cannot, however, see the nature of painfulness under the microscope. There is as yet, nor will there likely be in the foreseeable future, a diagnostic test for pain. Nonetheless, there are ample reasons to presume that a state of chronic pain represents, like cancer and infection, a single core illness.

Most texts define chronic pain as that which persists beyond six months. That is certainly an inclusive and encompassing definition. Few would debate that pain of six months' duration constitutes chronic pain. The time value, however, is highly arbitrary, almost to the point of meaninglessness. Surely the patient who suffers incessant pain should not have to wait six months before being accorded a diagnosis!

Let's look at some specific examples. A muscular sprain or overuse injury usually resolves within a few days or weeks at the most. A more severe injury, such as occurs to the ligaments in an ankle sprain, may last several weeks or even a few months. Shingles usually lasts four to six weeks. A ruptured disc in the lumbar spine may cause persistent pain, but if the patient continues to hurt for anything approaching six months, surgery is warranted, and in that case recovery is usually achieved in a short while.

The time value of six months is much too long, but it is useful simply because it recognizes that *almost any painful condition should resolve within a measurable time frame.* This offers a new dimension to our definition—chronic pain is that which persists beyond the anticipated time of recovery. It begins when the patient should be getting better but isn't. This is admittedly a very subjective definition. The lay person will be annoyed by its imprecision, but every physician knows exactly what I am talking about.

Let's fast-forward to another idea, one which is the central theme of this book. Chronic pain, I will suggest, is the product of the mind, and it begins at that point in time when pain becomes a cerebral rather than a somatic experience. When pain persists longer than it should, beyond accountability, a variety of seemingly unrelated things happen, and they usually occur within a rather short interval. Appetite changes. Sleep becomes disordered and nonrestorative.

Exhaustion and fatigue overwhelm. Memory is impaired, and the very act of thought disordered into persistent ruminations about pain. Mood is affected with fractiousness, irritability, and depression. All of these are a product of a mind in disarray, and they are the cardinal symptoms and identifiers of chronic pain. Now we can really get our teeth into a definition. Chronic pain is a state of pain characterized by destruction of the very architecture of fundamental existence. With that in mind, let's look at a few examples of what is and what is not chronic pain.

The migraine headache can be extraordinarily painful. As every migraineur (one who suffers migraine) knows, it can be a devastating experience, attended by disordered sleep, loss of appetite, and sometimes profound changes in mood. These, certainly, are the symptoms of chronic pain, but in the migraineur they last but a few hours or a few days at the most. Migraine is a disease of intermittent painfulness. It is not chronic pain. That is a disorder of incessant painfulness (there are exceptions, but these will be addressed later).

Rheumatoid arthritis is an inflammatory disease of the joints. It is a crippling and sometimes even mutilating disease, and it can be very painful, but it is not chronic pain. Most rheumatoids live useful and effective lives. They do not want for sleep, appetite, or good humor.

Shingles can be a dreadful disease. It generates severe pain that lasts for weeks. During that interval, the patient experiences all the symptoms of chronic pain. Sleep is disordered with frequent painful awakenings. Appetite is diminished. Food loses its flavor. Emotions are disordered with irritability and despondency. The architecture of a useful and happy existence is destroyed. Does this mean that the patient with shingles suffers chronic pain? Perhaps, but probably not—because although he may lose sleep, energy, and appetite, he does not lose hope. He can be told that his painful experience will be self-limited and that with time he will get well. Compare with fibromyalgia and tension headache. Victims of those disorders cannot be told that they will spontaneously recover. It is the lack of hope, perhaps more than anything else, that defines chronic pain.

Shingles, destructive though it is, is not chronic pain, but it may evolve into that disorder. Just as a muscular sprain may evolve into fibromyalgia, and migraine into tension headache, shingles may lead into chronic pain in the form of post-herpetic neuralgia. Perhaps in no other illness can the progression of acute into chronic pain be so clearly demarcated. It occurs at that point in time when the infection is arrested and the rash disappears, but the pain continues—when the patient should be getting better but isn't. This is also the point at which pain loses certain pathologic accountability. The nerves, so inflamed and dysfunctional during the acute interval, have regained their integrity. They show no abnormality to even the most discriminating tests of their structure and function, and yet they continue to generate a pain which will last a lifetime.

Let's compare pain, as I will do often in this book, with other experiences. That of grief is a good place to start. With the loss of a loved one, we mourn. We are saddened and tearful, sleep-deprived, anxious, and subject to strange imaginings and often a sense of guilt. These, it bears emphasis, are expected, even normal behaviors (just as the pain of shingles is an expected and normal behavior). Grief, like most pain, is typically a self-limited experience. With time, it goes away. Occasionally it persists though, and when grief lasts longer than it should (and again we are forced to meet an uncertain time frame), the experience of sadness is no longer just grief. It is depression, and that is a disease. Grief may evolve into depression just as shingles may evolve into post-herpetic neuralgia. The analogy is more than apt.

Pain begins in the body with corporal injury, usually a random and accountable event. When it persists beyond accountability, it becomes a mind-dominant experience associated with a stunning variety of behavioral effects. These are the symptoms of chronic pain, and it is their study, quite as much as that of pain itself, that will allow us some understanding of the disease. It is quite difficult, most of the time, to say exactly *when* chronic pain begins. We have but modest understanding of exactly *how* it happens, but we can see, with great clarity of vision if we but try, just *why* it happens.

CHAPTER THREE

Identifiers and Risk Factors

A curious attribute of patients with chronic pain is their tendency to develop different expressions of their illness. They often suffer multiple painful diseases simultaneously. For example, the concurrence of the irritable bowel syndrome, fibromyalgia, and tension headache in a single patient is not uncommon at all! There is an enormous overlap among the different syndromes of pain. Rather few of them are clear-cut, distinct entities. They often coexist with one another, and they often evolve one into another.

A woman with a ruptured lumbar disc comes to surgery but fails to recover. Her low back pain continues. With time, she begins to experience pain in her mid-back and shoulders. No cause can be found. She is accorded the diagnosis of fibromyalgia. Further along, she begins to suffer chronic pain in the neck and head. She is then accorded the diagnosis of tension headache. This type of scenario plays out again and again. It is the destiny of many patients to suffer not just one, but multiple painful diseases. The reader with chronic pain will, I am sure, attest to the validity of this statement. What does it all mean? Does it represent just a run of bad luck in the unprivileged few, or does it occur by some biologic design?

We are not going to understand the nature of chronic pain by dissecting and analyzing its component parts. The study of painful disorders such as headache and fibromyalgia, the delineation of their clinical boundaries and the features that make them distinct illnesses, is certainly a worthy endeavor, but it is not the object of this book. The most remarkable feature of these and other painful diseases is not how different they are from each other, but rather how much alike they really are. There is a master template, a biologic design, which dictates their several behaviors. Therefore, we will abandon the notion that painful patients suffer several different diseases and say simply that a singular characteristic of chronic pain is its capacity to spread beyond the site of its origin. This is not nearly as fanciful as it might seem at first pass.

The pain of acute cardiac injury, a heart attack, is often felt in the arm or in the jaw. That of pancreas inflammation may be felt in the back and that of gallbladder disease in the shoulder. All of these represent, of course, the *referral* of pain. It should take no leap of imagination to accept that chronic pain may also be referred. It moves and spreads, almost invariably, to other body parts and in a very unique manner.

Chronic pain is usually bilateral pain. This is one of many strange characteristics of the disorder. Pain which begins with injury on one side of the body gradually progresses to the opposite side, often in the fashion of a mirror image. For example, the pain of fibromyalgia, at its onset, is usually predominant in one side of the back, neck, or shoulder. With the passage of time, it invariably strikes the other side. Migraine is, by definition, a disease of unilateral pain, with headache confined to the left or right side. As migraine evolves into chronic pain, that which we know as tension headaches, pain spreads to the opposite side. Reflex sympathetic dystrophy is a painful disease associated with very dramatic stigmata. The painful limb becomes cold and atrophic. As the disease progresses, these same stigmata sometime appear inexplicably in the opposite, undamaged extremity! Strange as it may seem, chronic pain is often a *symmetric* disease. Many patients, particularly those whose pain is long-standing, state categorically that they simply hurt all over. The migration of pain and its extension to other body parts is an identifier of the disease.

Patients with chronic pain are invariably sleep-disturbed. We all know the restless sleep that occurs with injury and illness, but that of chronic pain is unique in its variety of strange expressions. Some patients actually experience hypersomnia—they sleep too much. Much more often they hardly sleep at all. Pain worsens at night and attempts to sleep actually aggravate pain. The painful dread the coming of the night. They are subject to nocturnal tremors such as myoclonus and restless legs. The normal physiologic pattern of alternating light and deep sleep is lost. As a result, sleep in the painful is nonrestorative—and often dreamless. Some patients suffer terminal sleep disturbance—that is sleep is initiated uneventfully, but painful awakenings occur early in the morning. Many take hot baths in the middle of the night in an effort to relieve their pain. A very curious feature is the occurrence of nocturia, awakenings throughout the night to empty the bladder. The association of nocturia with chronic pain is not widely recognized, but it is quite common. Disordered sleep is a certain identifier of chronic pain.

Chronic pain causes profound alterations in appetite and weight. This produces one of the most visible identifiers of the disease, for painful patients are often very obese. Some (chronic pain is a disease of contrasting effects) experience anorexia with disgust for food, and weight loss may occur. More often there is weight gain, often of astonishing proportions—one hundred pounds or more. It is convenient and perhaps logical to ascribe obesity to the inactivity and perhaps the boredom imposed by chronic pain. The seeking of gratification in the form of food when no other gratifications are available is an understandable behavior, but to ascribe weight gain simply to inactivity, boredom, or gratification-seeking is to miss the mark. In the old days when we put patients with tuberculosis on absolute bed rest for months at a time (certainly a boring and gratificationless existence), they would gain weight on the order of ten or fifteen pounds, rarely more than that. We can't blame weight gain on inactivity. It is due to something more fundamental. This is evident in the strange disorders of appetite that are seen so frequently. Many patients experience bizarre cravings, especially for sweets. In others, there are intervals of food gorging alternating with intervals of no desire for food at all. The simplest act of our existence, the maintenance of metabolic energy by the ingestion of food, is highly disordered in patients with chronic pain. It doesn't happen in everyone, only most. Disordered appetite—and obesity—is an identifier of chronic pain.

The object of caloric intake is the maintenance of metabolic energy. Patients with chronic pain, although often endowed with a surfeit of calories, want for energy—metabolic, physical, emotional, and even sexual. They uniformly experience diminished libido. Few are sexually active. Fatigue is a cardinal identifier of chronic pain. Indeed, the syndromes of chronic fatigue and chronic pain are almost certainly one disease, perhaps reverse sides of the same coin.

The regulation of visceral activity and the circulation of the blood are the domain of that segment of the nervous system known as the autonomic. It is a subconscious, automatic system. It controls the motility of the intestines, the maintenance of blood pressure and cardiac output, and the distribution of blood to those body parts which most need it (the intestines when we eat, the brain when we think, and the bone when we break it). These are highly adaptive behaviors and they represent the workings of a healthy and efficient autonomic nervous system. In patients with chronic pain, however, the autonomic nervous system is anything but healthy. It loses its harmony—thus bladder voidings which should occur in the day occur at night. Nocturia is but one expression of autonomic disorder in chronic pain. In the irritable bowel syndrome, the harmonious and synergistic movements of the intestine are disordered into wild swings of amplitude, introducing into consciousness painful and explosive diarrhea. Migraine itself is a form of autonomic dysfunction. Regional blood flow is highly disordered with swings in blood vessel tone. There are intervals of vasoconstriction with cerebral ischemia followed by vasodilatation and headache.

With an acute injury, such as the fracture of a bone, blood flow to the affected part is increased. Metabolic activity and the repara-tive process are thus enhanced. In patients with chronic pain, the opposite happens. This is most evident in reflex sympathetic dystrophy. Blood flow is diminished, and the painful part becomes cold. We tend to view reflex sympathetic dystrophy, which is a very dramatic illness, as a discrete medical entity, but it is not. There is enormous overlap among painful diseases, and most forms of chronic pain are associated with diminished blood flow. Whereas the acutely painful injury is warm to the touch, the chronically painful one is cool.

There is yet another identifier of chronic pain, and that is the phenomenon of *hyperpathia*. The perception of pain is malevolently enhanced. The most trivial stimulus, such as touching with a tissue or even blowing across the injured area, will generate pain. Hyperpathia is most common in reflex sympathetic dystrophy, but it is by no means confined to that disorder. Migraine (not a true chronic pain, but so intimately related to the disease that I will refer to it often) is associated with hyperpathia. The migraineur often reports, "My scalp is sore to touch." The patient with fibromyalgia experiences hyperpathia in the form of trigger points, localized areas that are extremely sensitive and painful to palpation. The patient with chronic pelvic pain often experiences hyperpathia in the form of dyspareunia, painful sexual intercourse.

The highest acts of our consciousness—those of mood, temperament, and thought—are disordered in chronic pain. Cognition, and its companion, memory, are impaired. Patients become forgetful and distractible. Simple intellectual tasks become labors. This effect is well-recognized in at least one painful disease—fibromyalgia. It is known, memorably, as the mind fog of that disease. Mind fog is by no means unique to fibromyalgia. It is an attribute of chronic pain across the board. On formal testing of intelligence and memory, painful patients often show impairments, sometimes approaching those seen in dementia.

Unremitting pain becomes unremitting thought—an obsession. Thought may be bent into delusions. "There is a hot poker in my back." "My skull is being forced down into my spine." The physician will certainly recognize that descriptions such as these are common in the chronically painful, but that they are never heard from patients with acute pain. Delusional thought is common, perhaps understandably, in those who suffer that form of pain which is most rich in symbolic and psychologic authority. Genital pain is frequently described with highly dramatic and bizarre sexual imagery.

There is another form of thought warp, known as conversion reaction, that occurs occasionally in painful patients. It is character-ized by a sudden loss of neurologic function

The identifiers of pain . . . are, in many patients, present long before pain appears.

such as paralysis, blindness, or loss of sensa-tion. It has no biologic accountability. So far as we know, patients with conversion reaction are capable of movement and vision, but they think they are not. Conversion is by no means confined to people with chronic pain, but it does occur with more than expected frequency in that disease. Thus, complaints such as "my legs hurt so much that they are paralyzed," and "I can't feel my husband in me anymore" are not uncommon at all.

Mood and temperament are altered, and as is often the case with chronic pain, in very contrasting ways. Some patients become restless, wired, and hyperactive. Sleep is disturbed not only by pain, but also by thought racing and an inability to turn off the mind. The majority, however, become listless, apathetic, tearful, and despondent with ruminations of hopelessness and sometimes of suicide. The very structure of personality is fractured. "I am just not the same person I was before I got sick." Painful patients say this a lot. And so do patients with depression. Those with other chronic illnesses, even cancer, rarely say it.

Depression is the most common psychiatric disease. Its inci-dence in debilitating illnesses such as stroke is, understandably, quite high. It is staggeringly high in chronic pain. The coexis-tence of depression and pain has been the object of study—and confusion—for many years. The identifiers of chronic pain are disordered sleep, appetite, energy, cognition, mood, and thought.

These are also the identifiers of major depression. This has led inevitably to the conclusion that depression and pain are the same illness. The two diseases fit the same template. At times, they are indistinguishable.

An important feature of both pain and depression is their frequent association with drug abuse. Patients become dependent and sometimes addicted to sleeping pills, tranquilizers, and opiates. Many become addicted to alcohol (a temporarily effective treatment for both pain and depression). Every psychiatrist knows that abstinence from drugs of abuse is fundamental to the successful treatment of depression. This is not an easy achievement, even in the best of circumstances. It is well nigh impossible in painful patients, for addictive, painkilling drugs are the only ones that give any relief.

There is certainly more to chronic pain than the experience of corporal discomfort. It is a vastly complex illness, associated with a variety of behavioral effects. These occur with great regularity. Why? Is it simply *because* pain is so commanding and destructive that it obliterates useful existence? Let's address the issue of causality. The painful can't sleep *because* pain keeps them awake. They gain weight *because* there is nothing else to do but eat. They are fatigued *because* they are constantly fighting pain. They are drug-dependent *because* of pain. They are depressed *because* of pain. These conclusions are commonsensical and logical, but they are almost certainly wrong. This is evident on even the most cursory examination. Why do the many and varied behaviors (identifiers) of pain appear with such consistency and utter predictability? Again, let's compare pain with other diseases. Cancer and stroke are very destructive illnesses. They leave quite a large wake, but in neither disease are the behavioral symptoms as profound, varied, and yet predictable as those which occur with chronic pain.

Now we come to the very heart of the matter. The identifiers of pain—the disordered sleep, appetite, energy, thought, mood, and even the drug dependency that we ascribe to the effects of the disease—are, in many patients, *present long before pain appears*. They are not the product of pain. They are antecedent to it. This observation, which is central to any understanding of chronic pain, has not received the attention it deserves. Nonetheless, readers with chronic pain will surely recognize its validity. Let's take them one by one.

Many patients suffer insomnia long before the advent of pain. Most want for sleep, but some are sleep-needless—four or five hours will do just fine (again, chronic pain is a disease of curious contrasts). The frequency of disordered sleep in patients who develop chronic pain is probably greater than 50 percent. In a sense, sleeplessness is a predictor for the development of the disease. Most physicians aren't aware of this, but rheumatologists certainly are. They know well that insomnia frequently heralds the onset of fibromyalgia. It also, without question, heralds other painful diseases. Remarkably, so do restless legs. Many experience the movement disorder for years before the advent of pain.

Many patients are appetite-disordered and obese long before they become painful. They are often subject to extreme weight fluctuations. They diet successfully, often many times, but they are unable to sustain weight loss. Not a few experience intervals of anorexia punctuated by food gorgings and purgings, the anorexia-bulimia syndrome.

A significant number of patients with chronic pain have suffered some cerebral injury along the way. This may be dramatic, as occurs with meningitis, epilepsy, or head injury. More often it is subtle, such as the minor cognitive impairment that appears after coronary bypass surgery or in the elderly who suffer cerebral vascular disease. Painful patients are thought- and memory-impaired, not just after the illness, but before it. Stated another way, painfulness often appears after stroke, closed-head injury, or coronary bypass surgery.

The incidence of depressive illness in those who develop pain is astonishing in its frequency. The majority of people who suffer chronic pain have experienced a depression of severity sufficient to warrant drug treatment, and in some cases even shock therapy, long before the onset of painfulness. Many offer a history of recurrent depressive interludes. A history of depression is, without question, the most common predictor of chronic pain.

Some patients experience throughout their lives a pattern of mood and behavior that is quite contrary to depression. They are wired, hyperactive, and sleep-needless, capable of doing two or three things at once. Against what we might expect, many who develop chronic pain were highly successful in their life endeavors. They are almost manic in their supercharged, mind-busy intellectual and physical energy.

There is as yet another antecedent of chronic pain, and with it we come almost full circle. A great number of victims have experienced drug abuse before the onset of their painfulness. The incidence of alcoholism is particularly high. Strangely, a lot of them have entered recovery and are abstinent until pain invites the reappearance of the behavior.

People do not become sleep- and appetite-disordered, depressed, or drug-dependent *because* they have pain. In most cases, these behaviors, at least some of them, were present and operative long before pain began. They occur with such frequency that they can justifiably be considered risk factors. They are as much predictors of pain as high cholesterol is a predictor of heart disease and smoking a predictor of lung cancer.

There is yet one more important risk factor for pain, and it must be mentioned although it is unpleasant to do so. Childhood neglect and abuse, particularly sexual abuse, are common experiences among those who develop pain. The association between childhood abuse and chronic pain is well known to psychiatrists. Few other physicians are as aware. The subject is rarely broached in interview. It is a taboo, and most physicians, fearful of giving offense (or opening a can of worms), avoid the interrogation, but the issue is there whether we choose to look at it or not.

The role of sexual abuse in the generation of pain will be addressed in detail many times in this book, but I will offer a foretaste. It often begins in the preteen years when an immature mind has difficulty reacting to such a profound stress. Many victims, perhaps most, accommodate to the experience and lead useful, if not always emotionally comfortable lives. In some, however, emotional and biologic development is deformed, permanently, into the total disintegration of the architecture of a meaningful existence. They suffer, throughout their lives, irregular sleep and appetite, periods of thought racing hyperactivity, anxiety, and interludes of depression. Mood and behaviors swing widely from one extreme to another. Suicide attempts are not uncommon, nor is conversion reaction. Drug abuse and addiction occur with unseeming frequency. Even the structure of personality is fractured. Abused children sometimes suffer multiple personality disorder.

Some psychiatrists believe that the pain which accrues to those who have suffered sexual abuse is a form of symbolic behavior. The victims express their emotional hurt as corporal pain. Most are female, and not a few suffer unaccountable pelvic pain. It requires little imagination to accept that particular symptom as a symbol. Perhaps symbolic also is another attribute of the abused. They are often obese. Symbolically, they make themselves unattractive to men.

We can, without difficulty, extend the idea of symbolism even to the non-abused. Depressives certainly know emotional hurt and so do alcoholics (that is why they drink!). The inability to sleep and the inability to control weight are certainly emotional experiences. And so, God knows, is the experience of childhood sexual abuse. Is chronic pain, particularly that of uncertain origin (and most chronic pains are of uncertain origin), a psychologic disorder?

I give many court depositions. In the course of each of them, I am asked—and this is invariable—"Is this person's pain some kind of psychologic illness?" A cruel question perhaps, but it is really no different from that of the painful patient who says, "I am a *strong* person. Why has this happened to me?"

CHAPTER FOUR

Mind-Soul Disease

A ll cultures have recognized a world of spirit removed from corporal existence. The Greeks were perhaps the first to codify spirit or soul as inherent to humanness and unique to each individual. The Judeo-Christian belief extended the concept of soul as man's link with God, thereby giving it the attributes of empowerment, responsibility, and accountability. The body decayed, but the soul lived forever. Soul and flesh were different entities. Our cultural heritage has accorded us a legacy, that of a mind-body dichotomy. The body has gradually yielded its secrets to scientific inquiry. Human dissection led to the understanding of organ systems, but the mind-soul did not yield its secrets so easily. Through the ages, deviant and unaccountable behaviors including madness, melancholy (depression), epilepsy, and we can be certain, chronic pain, were ascribed to an unempowered mind-soul. The advent of neuroscience and molecular biology, appearing only in the past few decades, has begun to disassemble the mind-body dichotomy. It remains with us, however, expressing itself in many, mostly nefarious ways. We continue to ascribe unaccountable diseases to the mind. This is not an entirely bad conceit—it is just that we view the mind in this context as an organ of character, will, and empowerment, somehow different and beyond the laws of biology which govern the rest of the body. For much too long, psychiatric disease was thought to be due to spiritual weakness.

Clinical medicine became a truly scientific discipline in the first half of the twentieth century. The discovery of the x-ray, the electrocardiogram, and the increasing refinement of biochemistry led to the understanding of the biologic (organic) diseases. These advances, however, afforded no insight into the nature of psychiatric illness, and for the first half of the twentieth century, mind-soul disease languished as a medical backwater, an object of theory but little in the way of scientific substance. Among the theories was one relating to the explanation of diseases, such as chronic pain, which appeared to occur at the interface of the mind and the body. Many painful patients lacked defining pathology to account for their complaints. Their illness was ascribed, conveniently, to the mind-soul. They suffered *psychosomatic* illness. (That particular word certainly pays homage to the mind-body dichotomy.) It was presumed that in those with psychosomatic illness, the organ systems were intact and operative but worked in a dysfunctional manner. The irritable bowel syndrome was due to dyssynergic movements of the stomach and bowels. Tension headache was due to sustained muscle contracture over the neck and scalp. Fibromyalgia was the same, dysfunctional contractions of the muscles adjacent to the spine. These and kindred diseases came to be recognized as *functional* disorders (the term psychosomatic, roughly equivalent to functional, has largely disappeared from the lexicon). Functional diseases were ascribed to emotion, and they were identified with neurologic descriptors—*irritable* bowel, *spastic* colon, *nervous* stomach, *tension* headache. These are not bad descriptors, but hardly good ones. There are worse. Conversion reaction (presumably a functional disease) used to be called hysteria, from the Greek, *hystera*, the uterus. Thus, functional disease represented the subjugation of the body to those systems endowed with the greatest psychologic and symbolic authority, the mind and the genital organs.

Functional disease was a medical wastebasket. It was that disease, or rather large group of diseases, for which physicians had no coherent explanation. For quite a long while, all diseases of uncertain origin, even peptic ulcer and colitis, were suspected to be psychosomatic in origin. There are a lot fewer functional diseases today because, as medicine has become more refined, the unknown has become the known. Peptic ulcer is no longer a functional disease. We now know that it is due to a bacterial infection. But the idea that a weak body may be due to a weak mind remains with us. We still have tension headaches and irritable bowels, and we still have conversion reactions. Our understanding of these diseases has advanced but little.

Unfortunately, functional disease is a second-class illness. We, as physicians and caregivers, treat patients with diseases such as cancer and heart attack with scientific discipline and compassionate, sensitive care. Do we always do this for the patient who suffers fibromyalgia or tension headaches? Painful readers will certainly be aware that they are the object, sometimes subtly and sometimes not, of disparagement.

Disability insurers certainly disparage those with functional diseases. If pain is due to an organic lesion, disability benefits are provided. In the absence of organic pathology, pain is suspect and recompense often denied. Managed care organizations also recognize, to their profit, a difference between diseases of the mind and those the body. Migraine has no certain pathologic accountability and is, therefore, a mind-soul disease. For this reason, insurers often deny or limit the quantity of the very effective and expensive drugs we currently posses for the treatment of migraine. Viagra is a marvelously effective drug for the correction of impotence, and if the patient can demonstrate a biologic cause for his impotence, be this multiple sclerosis, spinal injury, or diabetes, a quantity— perhaps a chaste quantity—can be provided. But if the cause of impotence is indeterminate, if it is *psychogenic*, a mind-soul disease, its treatment is the patient's responsibility and not the insurer's.

Managed care is a convenient whipping boy. Economic circumstances have made it the anvil on which medical practice is forged, and if it takes a little heat, so be it. But our insurance and medical practice really represent nothing more than our societal attitudes, and society still looks askance at the patient with unaccountable behaviors and unaccountable pains. If the etiology and pathology of a disease cannot be measured or quantified, it is suspect. A sad commentary, but reflective of two thousand years of belief in a mind-body dichotomy.

Functional disease, we used to believe, did not obey the dictates of biologic law. It came from higher authority, that of the mind-soul and its unempowerment. It was due to a flaw in spirit and character. Unaccountable diseases and unaccountable behaviors were the product of weakness. The disease was the patient's responsibility, not the physician's.

The entirety of human functioning . . . is dictated by the release and uptake of neurotransmitters. It is disorder in this system that is responsible for most of humankind's diseases.

One of the disorders for which we held the patient responsible was alcoholism. There was no biologic explanation for substance abuse. We viewed the behavior as a sign of characterologic weakness. We observed, or thought we observed, that alcoholics had a personality type characterized by passivity and dependency. The males seemed to marry strong dominant women who could accommodate to their habit and perhaps even enjoy the opportunities for control it afforded. At the time it all seemed to fit. Alcoholism was a disorder of those attributes that we might define as will, morality, and discipline. The alcoholic was a weak person lacking that essential core of strength that allowed him to resist temptation. This was, believe it or not, the science of the day.

Then, a revolution—breathtaking in its simplicity—occurred in our thinking about alcoholism. Thoughtful physicians noted the strikingly positive family history of the behavior with the genetic pedigree finding expression even in children adopted into non-alcoholic families. This, and other discoveries, led to the understanding that alcoholism was not a disorder of character or personality, but rather was a biologic, genetically acquired disease, albeit one with unattractive social behaviors. When the unpleasant attributes of the alcoholic's behavior were removed from social judgment, however, and studied simply for what they were, the phenomenology of an illness, rational criteria for diagnosis emerged. Forty years ago the alcoholic was a weak person and treated as such—with derision. Today he is simply a person with a disease, like hypertension or diabetes, and treatment at a drug abuse center can be very effective.

I will write shortly about the incredible drugs that we possess for the treatment of mind-soul disorders. We do not yet, however, have a drug for substance abuse. Therefore, for its treatment, we employ the mind-body dichotomy, the struggle between flesh and spirit, between empowerment and weakness. "I have friends who love me. God loves me. I am worthy" (Empowerment). "I have been overtaken by an evil, alcohol" (Weakness). "I will overcome this" (Struggle). It is a pretty good treatment, really the only effective treatment we have for substance abuse. But some day, perhaps in the not-too-distant future, this form of therapy will be of historic interest only, for we will certainly find a drug with which to treat addiction. Behavior is biology. It is not a struggle between strength and weakness.

Spiritual empowerment is certainly a worthy treatment modality. It can be employed not only for substance abuse but also chronic pain, depression, and really just about any other disease. Let's be aware, however, that spiritual empowerment is a biologic as well as an emotional experience. When our spirits are happy, those chemicals within our brain which control the entirety of our behavior are happy also, working energy-efficiently, unconfused about which routing to take.

Nerve cells, called neurons, communicate with each other by the release of a chemical known as a neurotransmitter from one and its uptake by another. Some of these neurotransmitters—serotonin and noradrenaline—have already been mentioned. Others will be shortly. Brain cells are almost infinite in their number and their variety. The variety of neurotransmitters, however, is surprisingly modest. They number only a few hundred at most. Thus brain cells share neurotransmitters in a very interactive dynamic. There are many cells to one neurotransmitter and very probably many neurotransmitters to one cell. The entirety of human functioning, from the circulation of the blood, to the highest acts of our consciousness, our intelligence and our behavior, are dictated by the release and uptake of neurotransmitters. It is disorder in this system that is responsible for most of humankind's diseases. These include, to mention but a few at random, depression, schizophrenia, substance abuse, epilepsy, migraine, suicide, high blood pressure, impotence, and, almost certainly, chronic pain. The infectious, neoplastic, and degenerative diseases, all organic diseases associated with tissue destruction, are terrible scourges, but their destructiveness pales next to that of diseases engendered by abnormal release and uptake of neurotransmitters.

Neurons and their transmitters are concentrated in the brain, but they are also widely distributed throughout the body. The same chemicals which control thought, mood, and behavior also control the workings of the heart, lungs, blood vessels, intestines, and genitals. So much for the mind-body dichotomy. Behavior and biology are one. It has taken a long time to come to that conclusion.

The breathtaking advances of modern medicine really began to gather momentum at mid-twentieth century. It was a time of great discovery and excitement. Epidemic polio was being eradicated with a vaccine. Cortisone was available for the treatment of arthritis and asthma. Cardiac surgery for the repair of damaged heart valves was becoming routine. Dreadful and almost invariably lethal diseases such as meningitis and endocarditis were being cured within a few days by the administration of penicillin. There were, however, few such dramatic treatments for mind-soul disease. For epilepsy, there was Phenobarbital and Dilantin (good drugs and still used, but there are better ones). For delirium tremens (alcohol withdrawal), there was only Paraldehyde, a primitive and long-discarded drug. For chronic pain there were only the opiates, hardly the best form of therapy. For depression there were no drugs at all, only the brutal (but sometimes effective) electric shock therapy. For schizophrenia there was absolutely nothing—except institutionalization. Then there occurred, about 1960, a series of discoveries which led to the emergence of neuroscience and neuropharmacology, an evolution that we continue to witness to this day.

The first was the recognition that an extract of the *Rauwolfia* plant was helpful in the treatment of schizophrenia. The drug, now known as Reserpine, had been used for ages on the Indian subcontinent as a sedative. It was employed for that purpose in the West and was discovered, quite by accident, to diminish schizophrenic hallucinations. The use of the drug in the treatment of schizophrenia led to yet another discovery of at least equal significance—Reserpine lowered blood pressure! It rapidly became a mainstay in the treatment of hypertension and remained so for several decades. Medical science had stumbled upon a drug which alleviated the most profound mind-soul disease, schizophrenia, and was of equal utility in the treatment of an organic disease so easy of measurement that it could be diagnosed simply by the application of a blood pressure cuff. Reserpine was good for both the mind and the body.

The antihistamine drugs had arrived on the scene by 1960. One of the early ones, Benadryl, has stood the test of time and is still used. Others were discovered, but most were discarded as ineffective, a fate that fortunately escaped one of them, known generically as Chlorpromazine. During its clinical testing it was found, again quite by accident, to be anti-hallucinatory. It was the breakthrough drug in the treatment of schizophrenia, much better than Reserpine. We know it today as Thorazine.

A particular challenge at mid-century was finding an antibiotic for the treatment of tuberculosis, a disease against which penicillin was ineffective. An anti-tubercular drug, known as Isoniazide, was finally identified. It was another breakthrough drug. Vastly important in its own right, it led to a truly astonishing discovery. Physicians in tuberculosis sanitaria noticed that some of their patients on Isoniazide experienced a sense of euphoria and wellness. Isoniazide, an antibiotic, was, believe it or not, the first antidepressant drug! Minor adjustments in its chemical configuration resulted in a class of agents known as monoamine oxidase inhibitors. They were widely used not only for the treatment of depression, but also hypertension. They are useful even now for the treatment of Parkinson's disease. Medical science had found yet another drug effective in the treatment of both the mind and body.

The monamine oxidase inhibitors had some disconcerting effects. In occasional clinical circumstances they produced a catastrophic and often fatal rise in blood pressure. They were effective drugs in the treatment of depression, but they were dangerous. Better ones were needed, and they were discovered in short order—again by accident. Pharmacologists were manipulating the structure of the Thorazine molecule in an effort to find other anti-schizophrenic drugs. They found several (one of them, Stelazine, will be discussed shortly). In the course of their investigations they created a spin-off drug, one whose chemical configuration, known as tricyclic, differed only slightly from that of Thorazine. It turned out to be ineffective in schizophrenia, but it was very useful in the treatment of depression. The tricyclic drugs were better and certainly safer than the monamine oxidase inhibitors. They quickly became the primary treatment for depression and remained so until the advent of Prozac and its derivatives some twenty years later. Nonetheless, they are still in use. It was discovered early on that they could be effective in the treatment of chronic pain. They were the first non-opiate drug useful for that disorder, and we continue to use them to this day.

In the span of but a few years, physicians discovered the first drugs for schizophrenia, the first drugs for depression, the first drugs for hypertension, and the first drug for chronic pain. Looking back on it now, we can see that this was the beginning of the end of the era of psychosomatic and functional disease.

Migraine is a painful illness, but it is not usually life-threatening although, curiously, there is a higher than expected incidence of suicide among migraineurs. Migraine is a periodic disease. There are protracted intervals of wellness interrupted by sudden sieges of headache. These are often precipitated by certain triggers, some change in the environment, which incites misbehavior in the brain and its blood vessels. A cascade of events follows with, in sequence, nausea and vomiting, distortion of vision, and then head pain which, strangely, often goes away with sleep.

There are many triggers in migraine. Certain fragrances, those of perfumes or flowers, and certain foods, chocolate, cheese, and wine, may cause headache. Menstruation often does, but it is emotional stress, a change in the psychologic environment, that is the most common trigger. Does this mean that migraine is a functional illness? For a long time we thought so. We observed that migraineurs had personality structures characterized by inflexibility and compulsiveness. The rigidity of their personalities made them poorly tolerant of change and disorder, and these circumstances triggered migraine. Compare with alcoholism. We thought that was a disorder of passive-dependent personality.

Then came Sansert, the first drug really effective in the prevention of migraine. It influenced the release of the neurotransmitter serotonin. That chemical is widely distributed throughout the body. In the intestines and blood vessels, serotonin controls contractility and dilitation, and in the brain the functions of mood, appetite, sleep, and yes, the perception of pain. Thus a drug which affected the release of serotonin might temper migraine either by its action on the brain or the blood vessels. In the case of Sansert, it turned out to be blood vessels. That was an important discovery, but certainly no greater than the realization that a drug could prevent migraine without influencing personality or behavior at all. Sansert and the other drugs which followed were to read the obsequies for functional illness.

I will now present the case histories of two patients seen long ago. It was at a time when scientific medicine was addressing the issue of mind-soul disease and the effects, for good or bad, of the new pharmacy which had appeared on the scene and offered such promise, not just in the treatment of patients, but in the understanding of the fundamental nature of their illness.

During my internship, I cared for a young woman who was both mentally retarded and schizophrenic. She was admitted in transfer from a local institution because of some bizarre behaviors. We were told only that she was acting very strangely, and that her medical records would arrive the next day. She drew a crowd in short order. She was writhing slowly about in bed, her head and neck rotating from side to side. Her arms would occasionally

extend with serpentine movements, and her trunk and pelvis undu-
lated to and fro. She could stand with assistance, but the slow
movements of her body continued. She was mute save for occasional gutteral sounds as her tongue moved about in her mouth. She
was reactive and would attempt to obey simple commands, but her
efforts only worsened the movements. Everybody took a look at
her, from the crack neurologist on down the chain of command. He
pronounced this a case of hysteria, conversion reaction.

Conversion reaction, we continue to believe to this day, is a
functional illness. Intolerable emotional stress is *converted* into a
somatic symptom, most commonly blindness or paralysis. All of us
react to stress with varying degrees of efficiency. Sometimes, rather
than meeting it head-on, we employ psychologic defense mechanisms. There are many of them and most are maladaptive. A
common one is denial. A man who experiences recurrent chest pain
radiating to his left arm is faced with an enormous stressor, that of
potential heart disease and perhaps sudden death. He may accommodate to the unendurable by denying its existence and ignoring
his symptoms. This is by no means an uncommon behavior, and it
often occurs in persons of considerable intellectual and emotional
endowment. Conversion reaction, on the other hand, is thought to
be the most primitive psychologic defense mechanism. It is seen
most frequently in the uneducated and intellectually unempowered,
and not in those more favorably endowed.

There is something very curious about conversion. Many
patients with the disorder ultimately develop a recognizable neurologic illness, not infrequently multiple sclerosis. This inconvenient
observation aside, we continue to believe that conversion occurs
most frequently in patients whose psychologic and emotional
resources are limited. Such patients are unempowered and, therefore, cannot cope.

We presumed that some untoward encounter had entered our
young patient's awareness and, responding to it with limited
resources, she converted emotional stress into a somatic symptom,
a bizarre movement disorder. It all made some sense. Most (not all)
conversion reactions dissipate over a few days. We expected her to

recover. So we all signed on—conversion reaction it was.

The nurses found her dead in bed the following morning. The answer was not long in coming. Her medical records arrived, and we learned that her hallucinations had recently become more severe, and that she had been given a new drug called Stelazine. A little library work revealed several cases of dystonic movement disorders due to Stelazine.

Among the neurotransmitters in the brain is one called dopamine. Excessive dopamine activity is operative in the disease schizophrenia. The predominant symptom of the disorder, hallucinations, can be controlled by blocking dopamine activity in the brain. A group of drugs known as phenothiazines have the capacity to block dopamine release and uptake. These drugs, among them Thorazine, Stelazine, and Trilafon predictably diminish hallucinations in the schizophrenic. So far so good. Would that it should be so simple.

Most neurotransmitters are small, rather simple molecules—easily metabolized and readily available for the neural apparatus. Nature, in its thrift, finding such chemicals, employs them for multiple uses—in several sites for several functions. In that area of the brain known as the limbic system, dopamine is involved with the integrity of thought. In an adjacent area, the basal ganglia, dopamine is employed to control gait and the movements of the extremities. A common disorder of the basal ganglia, Parkinson's disease, is due to dopamine insufficiency and is associated with muscular rigidity and tremor. Parkinsonism is treated by the administration of dopamine and this can be very helpful in restoring the fluidity of movement, but a side effect of dopamine therapy is the development, occasionally, of hallucinations, an unwanted spillover of the agent into the limbic system. Conversely, the treatment of schizophrenia with dopamine blockade may produce parkinsonism. It may also produce other movement disorders including dystonia, a slow, writhing tremor of the head, trunk, and extremities.

My patient didn't have conversion reaction. One doesn't die of conversion reaction. She had dystonia, and one can die of that. She did not have a functional disease. She had an organic disease. Her illness was the product of pharmacy, not of spiritual unempower-ment. We had missed something that we didn't need to miss. Critical data was not available to us, and we had failed to obtain a proper medical history. It is the medical history, more than anything else, that is so necessary in treating the obscure illness.

There is no guarantee that the unfortunate woman's life might have been saved had her physicians been more diligent. Still, one wonders if the outcome might have been better if all of us, top dog on down, had not leapt so blithely and willingly into the presump-tion that she suffered functional disease because she was retarded and schizophrenic, that she was different and somehow weak. Bad things happen when physicians ascribe diseases to emotional and characterologic weakness. No patient has ever been cured, nor has the meaning of any illness been elucidated by blaming it on the victim.

Tension headache is the most common form of chronic pain. Its time-honored but unfortunate name suggests that it is the product of stress and unresolved conflict. Its victims are usually trapped in dysfunc-tional marriages, dysfunctional jobs, and dysfunctional relationships. They are unempowered. They cannot escape circumstances over which they have no control. Their frustration and despair produces tension—emotional tension in the mind or muscular tension in the neck and scalp (take your pick)—and pain.

Toward the end of my residency, I encountered yet another patient with tension headache. We entered her darkened room and found her well coifed and groomed, supine in bed, laid out as on a bier, a wet washcloth over her forehead, her diaphanous gown laid over the contours of her ample body. My mentor mumbled the introductions and proceeded with his inquiry into her chronic head pains. He quickly did his neurologic examination, assured himself that her cognition and memory were intact, her visual and other special senses were operative, and that her gait and station were normal. There were no pathologic reflexes and he knew, as did I, that the likelihood of an organic illness, a brain tumor, was remote. He requested some laboratory testing, and then wrote an order for

Amitriptyline, a new tricyclic antidepressant, to be given at bedtime. This surprised me a bit. We usually gave a tranquilizer and muscle relaxant such as Meprobamate (recently arrived on the scene and known then as Equanil) and maybe an analgesic. Instead, this time Amitriptyline—not a tranquilizer at all but an antidepressant—an entirely different order of drug. My professor circumlocuted an explanation, telling her that he believed there was a functional disconnection to the nerves of the scalp, and it was unlikely that she had a serious illness. Perhaps a new medicine would alleviate her condition, an unusually hopeful suggestion I thought.

He departed and left me to obtain the obligatory personal and social history. She was a voluble and demonstrative person and offered without hesitation the story of her life. She was in her forties and a hairdresser. She had been married and divorced three times. It was her custom to drink a couple of glasses of vodka each night. Without that sedative, she would be quite unable to sleep. She had been a lifelong insomniac and subject, she acknowledged, to occasional intervals of depression. "Three divorces will make you depressed," she emphasized. She grew up in a broken home, and her stepfather was abusive to her. I think she wanted to tell me more about it, but I chose not to pursue the issue. I felt I had enough data, and there was nothing to be gained by emptying the closet of skeletons.

I reported my discoveries and asked my mentor if we should request psychiatric consultation. He replied, practical as always, "There is no need to do that. We would just antagonize her with the suggestion, and psychotherapy probably wouldn't help her headaches anyway. It almost never does."

The following morning she reported the best night's sleep in many years (even without vodka) and told us that she had no headache at all. Years of headache, a single Amitriptyline pill, and it was gone. Her response, I have since learned, was a flash in the pan. Only rarely is there an immediate response to Amitriptyline. The drug usually takes a couple of weeks to kick in, but an overnight effect does occasionally occur. That knowledge would all come later, but at the time I was reveling in my teacher's skill.

"Why did you use Amitriptyline? She doesn't complain of depression. She complains of headaches. Amitriptyline certainly helped her, but why?"

"She is depressed. She just doesn't know it. Her headaches and insomnia are symptoms of depression. They are *depressive equivalents*."

This was a new idea, and at the time a very good one. Depression need not present itself as despondency and hopelessness. It may present as a somatic complaint, usually some sort of painfulness. The recognition of this fundamental truth was small change, perhaps, compared to the revolution that was occurring in cardiac surgery, infectious disease, and rheumatology, but nonetheless it was very significant. A functional disease, tension headache, responded well to an antidepressant drug. Were chronically painful patients simply suffering a masked depression? Was functional disease, painful disease, really a disorder of personality or unempowerment? Personality structure and character are ingrained, lifelong attributes. They are profoundly difficult to change. Depression, plenty complicated enough, but nonetheless an acquired illness, is much easier to treat. Could it be that simple? Could chronic pain be nothing more than unrecognized depression? Certainly a hopeful idea. The lady with tension headache was, I am sure, one of the first patients ever treated successfully for chronic pain by a tricyclic drug.

Alcoholism, migraine, conversion, and chronic pain (tension headache) have all been considered diseases of spiritual and emotional unempowerment and an inability to cope. The alcoholic could not cope with temptation. The patient with conversion could not cope with stress. The migraineur could not cope with change, and the patient with tension headache could not cope with life. This, it bears emphasis, was the thinking of the best minds in medicine a scant four decades ago. Old ideas die hard. Two thousand years of a belief in the mind-body dichotomy won't be easily chased away. Physicians and society at large still tend (perhaps in moments of our own spiritual and intellectual unempowerment) to disparage these patients. They are viewed as somehow less worthy than the patient with a heart attack, pneumonia, or appendicitis. Stated another way, the average general physician, if asked to list those diseases he or she was most comfortable and confident in treating, would place alcoholism, migraine, conversion, and chronic pain at the very bottom.

Still, things are better than they were forty years ago. Let's take a look at where we stand today with mind-soul disease. Substance abuse is recognized by nearly everyone as a biologic disease, in many cases genetically acquired. It is not yet really amenable to biologic (drug) therapy, but there are some beginnings. Wellbutrin, an antidepressant, actually diminishes nicotine craving. Migraine is certainly a biologic illness. We have excellent drugs, at least a half-dozen for the treatment of the acute migraine headache and a few more for the prevention of recurrence. Nonetheless not all patients respond, and migraine can be a very frustrating illness to treat. Even today, those who fail to respond to appropriate therapy are suspected of being somehow emotionally unempowered. Both depression and schizophrenia are now recognized as biologic disorders, highly amenable to therapy with the new pharmacy.

> *Two thousand years of a belief in the mind-body dichotomy won't be easily chased away. Physicians and society at large still tend . . . to disparage these patients.*

Conversion reaction, however, remains nearly as much an enigma as when it was described over a hundred years ago. It is the disease, above all others, that we still ascribe to emotional and intellectual unempowerment. That may be changing. Sophisticated instruments which assay the dynamic function of the mind have demonstrated that in the patient with hysteric blindness, the occipital lobes of the brain (the area concerned with the perception of vision) behave quite differently, physiologically, from the rest of the brain. We will someday, and perhaps soon, understand that conversion is a biologic disorder, just as are substance abuse, migraine, depression, and schizophrenia.

This brings us to chronic pain. Only recently have we recognized that its victims suffer a true disease. Compare with alcoholism. We recognized substance abuse as a disease decades before we accorded chronic pain that dignity. We have been forced, finally, to the acceptance that chronic pain is a disorder of biology. Its clinical behavior is stereotyped and predictable, a fundamental attribute of biologic disease, and it is highly amenable to biologic therapy in the form of pharmacy.

Astonishingly, there are well over one hundred drugs which have been proved or certainly will be proved to be effective in the treatment of pain. No other disease is as responsive to so many drugs. Let's compare again. There are a dozen or so drugs useful in the treatment of epilepsy and perhaps an equal number for schizophrenia. For depression and its variant, manic-depressive illness, there are some fifty drugs. And yet for pain, there are over a hundred! A remarkable fact—most of the drugs used in the treatment of epilepsy, schizophrenia, and depression offer relief from chronic pain. While there is no drug that works on every patient with pain, all of them work on some. Why do so many drugs of such vastly different clinical indications and pharmacologic properties relieve pain? We can only speculate, but there may be an answer.

I suggest that chronic pain may be the most profound experience that a human being can endure. No other disease is as destructive to the entirety of being—to both the mind and the body—as is chronic pain. No other is as pervasive in the variety of its effects on the way the human organism works. Sleep, appetite, energy, mood, thought, memory, blood flow, and the fundamental perception of sensation are all disordered. Stated simply, there are more neural systems in disarray in chronic pain than any other illness. This is the reason so many drugs are effective.

CHAPTER FIVE

Drugs for Pain

The drugs useful for pain are vast in number and variety, but they can be conveniently divided into groupings. Some are identified by a common chemical structure and others by a common mode of biochemical action. The most widely used grouping, however, is based on clinical indications, that is, which drug for which disease. Thus there are antidepressant, anticonvulsant (anti-epileptic), antipsychotic (anti-schizophrenic), and anxiolytic (anti-anxiety) drugs. The reader will be advised that the classification of drugs according to their clinical indication is highly arbitrary. The great majority of pharmaceuticals, and this will surely be evident in the pages which follow, have multiple indications. Most are effective in the treatment of many different diseases.

The most commonly used drugs for the treatment of chronic pain are known collectively as analgesic (anti-pain) drugs. They may be subdivided, in a manner which the expert reader will recognize as somewhat simplistic, into two subgroups. One consists of agents which relieve pain by diminishing inflammation, the body's response to injury. Aspirin and Tylenol are familiar to everyone. Their mode of action is the relief of inflammation. They work at the site of injury by diminishing the release of chemicals which incite the peripheral nerves to send the message of pain to the brain. Similar drugs, and of more recent development, are known as non-steroidal anti-inflammatory drugs (NSAID). These agents imitate the action of cortisone, a drug supreme in the treatment of inflammation, but they lack that drug's *steroidal* chemical configuration. They also lack at least some of the disturbing side effects of cortisone, and they are the most effective drugs available for the treatment of everyday pains.

The second group, the true analgesic drugs, has little if any anti-inflammatory activity. They do their work not at the site of the injury but within the brain where they alter the transmission of the painful signal. The lowest order of analgesic drugs is identified, for lack of a better word, as opiate-like. Among them are Darvon, Nubain, Stadol, and Ultram. They are not true opiates for they lack that chemical configuration, but nonetheless they stimulate opiate (endorphin) receptors and thereby diminish pain. They are all synthetically derived. Their development was the product of the quest to find the perfect drug, a non-addictive pain killer. Unfortunately, all of them carry the silent partner of agents which stimulate the endorphin system, the risk of addiction. The next order of drugs on the scale of potency are the true opiates, Codeine, Hydrocodone, Oxycodone, and Methadone (yes, the same Methadone that is used in the treatment of heroin addiction, but also an effective analgesic and probably under-used). They are usually given orally, and they are very effective in the relief of moderate to severe pain such as occurs post-operatively or with shingles or a fracture. They are often combined in a treatment form known as *polypharmacy* with other drugs in order to increase their effectiveness. Darvocet, Lorcet, Percocet, and most recently, Ultracet are combinations of opiate and opiate-like drugs with Tylenol. The suffix, -cet, derives from Acetaminophen, the generic name for Tylenol.

The last drugs and the highest on the scale of potency are Morphine, Dilaudid, and Demerol. So dominant and commanding is their ability to relieve pain that there is no real need to hybridize them with other agents. Nonetheless, one of them, Demerol, slightly less effective than the others, is most often prescribed in combination with a phenothiazine in a drug form known as Mepergan (a derivation from Meperidine, the generic for Demerol, and Phenergan, the proprietary for Promethazine).

Unlike drugs to be discussed soon, the opiates are themselves neurotransmitters. Their therapeutic effect requires no neuronal adjustment. They stimulate, without any intermediary process, those cells dedicated to the immediate relief of pain. They act quickly, and for the treatment of acute pain they are incomparable. Their side effects are modest and, although in extravagant doses they can produce respiratory depression, they are, in the hands of a competent physician, among the safest drugs in all of medicine. There is no pain that cannot be adequately relieved by opiates. However, the longer the pain lasts, the less effective the opiates become. The opiate-endorphin neurotransmitter system is an immediate response team, designed for prompt, short-term control of pain. After an interval of several days or perhaps a few weeks, the control of pain passes to other neural systems, those employing the neurotransmitters serotonin and noradrenaline. Opiates can certainly be helpful in the treatment of chronic pain, but their use is somewhat contrary to the laws of nature and for this reason, with the passage of time, it requires more and more opiate to relieve pain. This effect is known clinically as the phenomenon of *tolerance*.

The brain is a society of neurons, all working in a harmonious manner, subject to physiologic checks and balances. The long-term administration of opiates invigorates some members of that society by constantly bathing them in the neurotransmitter of their choice. In the absence of any physiologic restraint, they become dominant and dictatorial in their behavior. This effect is known clinically as the phenomenon of *addiction*. The opiates share with many other drugs (including barbiturates, tranquilizers, alcohol, nicotine, and caffeine) the capacity to invite, with their prolonged use, addiction and its attendant behaviors.

A word now about drug dependence and drug addiction. The former is very common; the latter in the large scheme of things, rather rare. Many patients are dependent upon pharmaceuticals— opiates, tranquilizers, and even antidepressants. The sudden cessation of these drugs in patients accustomed to taking them produces *withdrawal*, commonly anxiety, insomnia, tremors, abdominal cramps, and even seizures. Drug dependence implies an emotional and physical need for the agent, and the potential for withdrawal when the drug is terminated. The person with drug dependency needs a steady diet of their drug to function. A person addicted to a drug, however, requires more than a steady diet. Addiction is uncontrolled craving and the need for ever larger doses and more frequent administration. The risk of this development is, in the minds of most physicians, the greatest detriment to their use.

The use of opiates, how much and in which patient, is one of the most perplexing dilemmas facing the physician. Tolerance and dependency are almost invariable, and not a few patients, perhaps those genetically predisposed, develop addiction. As every physician knows, that disease can lead to extremes of behavior. Chronic pain is a cruel illness. Perhaps in no other disease is the quest for recovery balanced so unfavorably by the need to stay sick—in order to obtain disability benefits, win the lawsuit, or maintain the opiate habit.

Some physicians around the country, intelligent, far-sighted, and noble, have espoused the use of opiates in the treatment of chronic pain. They have emphasized that the benefits far outweigh the risks of addiction. Not many of their colleagues share the enthusiasm. Few physicians are comfortable prescribing opiates over the long term. The risk of addiction—and disciplinary action by state boards—weighs heavily on their minds. In the last analysis, however, these are peripheral issues (both occur only infrequently). The real issue is that the opiates are not very effective drugs. Perhaps surprisingly to those who have not shared the experience, most patients are not comfortable taking opiates. They don't like the stigma attached to the use of the drugs, nor do they enjoy the unnatural feeling state that attends their usage (it is only a minority of patients who experience a real sense of euphoria with opiates). Some painful patients on tricyclics and other drugs to be discussed shortly actually get well, or as close to well as one gets with a chronic illness. This doesn't happen with opiates. The patient on opiates doesn't get well. He just gets by.

Opiates can be helpful. They are, after all, supreme in the relief of pain. So we use them and sometimes liberally. We acknowledge their dangers and employ them with care. Unfortunately, it is much easier to use these drugs in persons whose source of pain can be demonstrated than in those who exhibit no painful pathology. It is ironic that society and medicine deem the use of opiates in painful patients dying from cancer a worthy and desirable form of treatment but deny others, equally painful without cancer, their benefits. We offer relief to those who are dying with pain but not those who are living with it. We are armed with drugs that do give pain relief. It is preposterous not to use them when we have to. But our social and medical attitudes weigh heavily on our treatment of painful patients and are an enormous encumbrance.

There is currently a very fashionable illness, analgesic rebound headache, perhaps known to many readers. Chronic headache (tension headache if we must) is an aggravating and painful condition, and people who suffer it seek relief with analgesics such as Ibuprofen or Tylenol. Sometimes they seek and are given stronger drugs such as Darvon or Ultram. Both of these have some addictive potential, but their occasional use by the painful patient hardly amounts to a state of depravity.

Chronic pain is a cruel illness. Perhaps in no other disease is the quest for recovery balanced so unfavorably by the need to stay sick—in order to obtain disability benefits, win the lawsuit, or maintain the opiate habit.

Rheumatoid arthritis is a chronically painful illness, and many patients with the disorder regularly use analgesic drugs for relief. This is recognized by all as appropriate therapy. No one would deny the use of Tylenol, Ibuprofen, or Darvon for such patients. Some neurologists, however, decry the use of these drugs in patients with chronic headache. That disease, unlike arthritis, has no pathologic accountability. It is, therefore, a mind-soul disorder. In a curious inversion of thought, almost magical thinking, they have come to ascribe recurring headaches to a rebound phenomena—the headache worsens as the analgesic drugs wear off. The idea is certainly not without merit. Many drugs, be they Ibuprofen, opiates, alcohol, or even caffeine, exhibit the rebound phenomena. The symptoms for which the drug is taken worsen as the drug wears off. However, to blame the symptoms on the drug is illogical. Would the pain of rheumatoid arthritis simply disappear if we quit using analgesics?

The mind-body dichotomy again. Corporal (organic) pain merits analgesic therapy. Mind (functional) pain does not. Our treatment strategies are skewed in opposite directions. Arthritic pain is certainly real pain. Does that mean that headache pain is not? "If you will just stop taking those pills, your headaches will get better." It rarely works. Blame the patient for the disease.

Let's go back to the lady with tension headaches and suppose, for the time being, that she had not been treated with Amitriptyline. She uses, as most patients with tension headaches do, over-the-counter analgesics. She encounters various physicians along the way and is given at different times drugs such as Darvon, Fiorinal, or Ultram. Our patient, at midlife, is functioning, but barely. She is chronically depressed and chronically painful. She carries the scars of childhood abuse, and she is alcohol and analgesic-dependent. She suffers an unfortunate but common life event. She slips and falls on her back, breaking one of the spinal vertebrae. The bone is compressed, accordion-like, and she suffers severe back pain. There is no definitive treatment for compression fractures. She will wear a back brace, limit weight-bearing, and endure the pain for several weeks. Tension headache may be a second class illness, but a vertebral compression fracture is certainly not. Her physician prescribes opiates, perhaps Hydrocodone or even Mepergan. This is appropriate—it would be unconscionable to deny the patient opiate therapy. She is instructed to take her drug every four hours as needed for pain. Her physician anticipates that within a week or two her pain will diminish and then can be controlled by lesser drugs. Our patient, however, fails to recover. A mind bent by childhood abuse, alcohol and drug dependency, and chronic depression lacks the resources to accommodate to a new and very painful injury. A couple of weeks later, she is still hurting, quite as badly as before. The frustrated physician has no recourse but to give more opiates. Barring some clinical miracle, she will continue to hurt, and her abnormal back x-ray, the legacy of a remote fracture, will be forever visible evidence of her pain and her need for opiates.

Now, let's introduce another element into this woman's story. We will say that she did receive Amitriptyline for her tension headaches, and that it was an effective drug. Her headaches disappeared, as did her depression. Her sleeplessness improved also, and she became less needful of vodka. Even though thrice married and divorced and childhood-abused, she achieves, with drug therapy, a life of some comfort and a sense of wellness. Then she falls and breaks her back. Would the outcome have been different? I believe so. I believe that there would be at least a reasonable chance that she would experience, as most people with compression fractures do, the gradual resolution of her pain and with it the need for opiates.

Chronic pain is the product of events and circumstances which were operative long before the disease becomes clinically manifest. The same can be said, of course, of many other diseases. The osteoporotic hip fracture is the result of years of lack of dietary calcium and of estrogen deficiency. The heart attack is the result of years of high cholesterol, hypertension, and smoking. The treatment of hip fracture entails surgical repair, but also the introduction of dietary calcium and drugs which restore the integrity of the bones. The treatment of heart disease often entails surgery, but also the introduction of drugs which restore the integrity of the arteries. Chronic pain can sometimes be treated by surgery, but the best treatment is the administration of drugs which restore the integrity of the mind.

The tricyclic drugs were the first non-opiate agents used for chronic pain. They are, by today's standards, rather primitive and unrefined drugs. They influence the action of many transmitters, but their predominant effect is to enhance the release of serotonin and noradrenaline. In their variety of effects, they are rather clumsy agents, but they are reasonably effective, and for many years they were all we had. They have a peculiar clinical attribute, as do most drugs which modify the serotonin and noradrenaline systems. They are slow in onset of action. It can be demonstrated in the laboratory that the agents provide an almost immediate release of transmitters, but their clinical effect, whether for the treatment of pain or depression, takes a couple of weeks to appear, as if some sort of rearrangement has to occur.

The efficacy of the tricyclic drugs in the treatment of pain was discovered early in their history. We presumed, for quite a long time, that chronic pain and depression were one in the same disease. Many patients with chronic pain are depressed, and many depressives suffer chronic pain. We would probably think that way still, but for the discovery of Prozac. That drug and its derivatives, Zoloft, Paxil, Celexa, and Luvox are identified by their mode of biochemical action. They are selective serotonin reuptake inhibitors (SSRI). They are clean drugs in that, unlike the tricyclics, they influence only a single neurotransmitter system, that of serotonin. They are vastly superior to the tricyclics in the treatment of depression. So great was the enthusiasm for them that it was presumed, without serious question, that they would be useful in relieving pain. They weren't—and this surprised everyone. Pain and depression are not the same disease, and it has taken a long time to figure that out.

> *Painfulness . . .*
> *was like*
> *depression in that*
> *it involved . . .*
> *the centralization*
> *of pain.*
> *Pain in the brain.*

The tricyclics are good for chronic pain. No one will contest that. But if we are not treating depression, what are we treating? The tricyclic drugs do have an analgesic effect. An experimental animal treated with tricyclics will require a greater stimulus threshold to exhibit a painful response than will an untreated animal. The effect is weak, however, probably no greater than that of aspirin, and yet the clinical efficacy of these drugs in painful patients is sometimes remarkable. The tricyclic effect began to make sense when we learned that there are brain centers which are actually dedicated to the control of pain. These analgesic centers are located in the brain base where they merge with nerve tracks carrying the painful signals from the body to the brain. They serve to filter and modulate the painful signal on the way to the upper brain and consciousness. They do this by employing not only serotonin but also noradrenaline. This effect, it turns out, is enhanced by the tricyclic drugs.

How did we discover that the tricyclics relieved pain? Originally, dumb luck. This often happens. The empiric use of a drug often precedes our understanding of why and how it works. The evolution of our knowledge of the brain's analgesic systems fit well, however, with what we observed clinically. A class of drugs, the tricyclics, propitiously abated a state of painfulness, and this affect was seemingly independent of any antidepressant activity. Painfulness wasn't depression, but it was like depression in that it involved, at least in part, a disorder of central nervous system neurotransmission. The *centralization* of pain. Pain in the brain. A profoundly important idea.

The tricyclics and the SSRIs have taken different paths. The SSRIs are useful in a variety of psychiatric disorders including depression, personality disorders, impulsivity, and phobias. Tricyclics aren't used much by psychiatrists now, but they remain useful for the treatment of pain and a few other disorders. They are still somewhat effective for depression and also for the treatment of insomnia. They are useful for preventing enuresis in children and, most curiously, they are effective in the treatment of cataplexy. That bizarre phenomenon occurs almost exclusively in persons with narcolepsy. They are subject, when startled, to a brief loss of muscle tone causing a sudden collapse without a loss of consciousness. It is a sort of dissociation, a suddenly asleep body and an awake mind. Thus a strange assembly of disorders—depression, pain, insomnia, bedwetting, and narcolepsy—are benefited by tricyclics. A remarkable range of diseases, they have one major attribute in common. They are all disorders of sleep. The tricyclics are useful, perhaps exclusively so, for sleep-disturbed patients, and painful patients are invariably sleep disturbed.

The restoration of sleep is a prime therapeutic goal in the treatment of pain. Rarely is there any diminution of pain until there is restoration of sleep. The tricyclics are pretty good, but not great, sleeping pills. There are much better ones, and these are often employed with tricyclics. Until recently, the most commonly used drugs belonged to a class of chemicals known as benzodiazepines of which Xanax and Valium are examples. These drugs act on the gamma-aminobutyric acid (GABA) neurotransmitter system. GABA neurons in the brain are inhibitory or, if you will, sedative neurons. GABA activity is augmented by the benzodiazepines and also by alcohol and barbiturates. These agents have in common that they are anxiolytic, soporific, and anticonvulsant (alcohol could be used for the treatment of convulsions; it is just inconvenient for that purpose). An unfortunate attribute of all these drugs is that they can induce both intoxication and addiction. They are useful but dangerous agents. The pharmaceutical industry has addressed this problem by creating a new class of drug of which Ambien and Sonata are examples. These are chemically different from benzodiazepines and barbiturates, but they stimulate GABA receptors in a similar manner. They are quick acting and of short duration and are relatively free of the addictive effects of the true benzodiazepines and other soporifics. They are splendid drugs for the treatment of insomnia, and it was presumed they would be helpful in the treatment of fibromyalgia and other painful disorders. Unfortunately it didn't work out that way. They are good for sleep, but they are not very good for pain. The true benzodiazepines are. They are very good indeed, and the best one (some physicians might debate this point) is the anticonvulsant Klonopin.

Anticonvulsants have long been used in the treatment of pain. Dilantin, discovered many years ago, was found early on to be helpful in the treatment of the pain of peripheral nerve injury. Epilepsy is due to irritability of nerve cells within the brain. The pain of neuritis is due to the irritability of peripheral nerves. The use of a single drug for both disorders made sense, and it worked pretty well. A later drug, known as Tegretol, worked even better, and it is still one of the cardinal drugs for the treatment of trigeminal neuralgia, a form of neuritic face pain.

There have been an abundance of new anticonvulsants to appear in recent years. The first was Depakote, followed by Neurontin, Lamactil, Topamax, and Keppra. Each are unique drugs with their own biochemical action. They were welcomed, not only because they were anticonvulsant, but because they held promise as another treatment for neuritic pain. As expected, they worked rather well for that disorder, but unexpectedly they also worked for migraine. Not only that, they were effective in the relief of many forms of chronic pain including fibromyalgia. They also had antidepressant properties, and this led to a remarkable discovery. The new anticonvulsants, all of them, are effective *mood stabilizers* in patients with bipolar, manic-depressive illness. They prevent the swings between emotional highs and lows that characterize the disorder. We have long known that Dilantin and Tegretol were modestly effective in the treatment of bipolar disease, but they were never used very much. Lithium, to be discussed shortly, was a much more effective drug, and it was the principal therapy for bipolar disease until the appearance of the new anticonvulsants. This brings us to a stunning observation, one of incontestable validity. Every drug that we employ for the treatment of manic-depression is also useful for the treatment of chronic pain. Is this merely coincidence?

Chronic pain is often associated with distinctive and identifiable psychiatric *comorbidities*. There is no doubt but that depression, substance abuse, and very probably bipolar illness have a high concordance with painfulness. So do appetite and sleep disorders. Are there other psychiatric illnesses which, in their complex clinical display, exhibit the symptom of chronic pain? Yes, almost certainly, and therein may lie the answer as to why so many drugs are useful in the treatment of painfulness.

Lithium is highly effective in the treatment of mania in the bipolar patient. It is also useful in the prevention of migraine. It has another peculiar attribute. It augments the antidepressant effects of tricyclics and SSRIs and is often combined with them (polypharmacy again) in the treatment of depression. Lithium can also be helpful in the treatment of chronic pain. The drug certainly doesn't work on everyone, but occasionally it works very well. Painfulness, insomnia, and restlessness dissipate—not completely (it is never complete)—but substantially and dramatically. In some patients Lithium just seems to go to the core of the disease. Many painful patients exhibit a high degree of restlessness, hyperactivity, and thought-racing. These behaviors are common in bipolar disease. As has been noted previously, a great number of painful patients were, before their illness, very active, creative, and achieving people.

Many manic, bipolar patients are achievers. It is easy for them. They have more energy than the rest of us. They are wired, little needful of sleep, and vastly successful in their life endeavors. Unfortunately, some of them develop chronic pain.

Thorazine and the related antipsychotic drugs are occasionally useful in the treatment of pain. A new group of drugs, known as atypical antipsychotics, are also finding usefulness. We come to another coincidence—those drugs which control thought can also control pain. Many patients who suffer chronic pain have been rendered thought and memory disordered by epilepsy, head injury, or stroke. We would anticipate that patients such as these would be the ones to respond to antipsychotic therapy, and that is, indeed, about the way it works out. Yet another psychiatric comorbidity to painfulness and a variety of drugs with which to treat it.

A caveat. It is much too simplistic to believe that some pains are due to depression, and if depression is treated the pain will go away. Or that some are due to substance abuse, and they too will go away when substance abuse is corrected. Or when epilepsy or manic-depressive illness is treated, the pain will go away. By no means does it always happen that way, but it does happen a lot. The conclusion is obvious. The same neuronal transmitter systems that are at the root of depression, substance abuse, bipolar illness, and certainly others lie also at the root of chronic pain.

Ritalin, a stimulant, is useful in the treatment of depression. Not surprisingly, it is sometimes helpful in the treatment of painfulness. It is also effective, of course, in the treatment of attention deficit disorder (ADD). That disease is typically associated with over-activity, restlessness, and mind racing, common behaviors in the painful patient. On the other side of the scale, ADD is a disease of inattention, and painful patients are often very attentive—to the point of obsession. In some regards, theirs obsessions parallel those of patients with obsessive-compulsive personality disorder (OCD). A disease of unremitting, obsessive thought, it is sometimes treated effectively by one of the newer tricyclics, Anafranil. It would be quite a stretch to say that painfulness might be symptomatic of ADD or OCD just because it has somewhat similar behaviors and similar responses to drugs, but still one wonders. The clinical spectrum of painfulness is broad indeed, and painful patients often exhibit fragments of many, very different neuropsychiatric disorders. That, I believe, will turn out to be quite important.

There are a vast number of drugs, of very different pharmacologic properties, that are useful in the treatment of pain. As is often the case in clinical medicine, no single drug is totally effective. Therefore we use them in combination. Once again, let's compare chronic pain—and its treatment—with other diseases. Endocrinologists employ polypharmacy in the treatment of diabetes. They can give insulin, or drugs which promote the secretion of insulin by the pancreas, or drugs which reduce the production of glucose by the liver, or drugs which enhance the uptake of glucose by the body's cells. Different drugs with different pharmacologic properties are used simultaneously. Cardiologists employ polypharmacy in the treatment of heart failure. They give diuretics to reduce blood volume, other drugs to relax arterial tension and reduce the work of the heart, others to stabilize the heart rhythm, and yet others to increase the force of cardiac contraction. The treatment of both diabetes and congestive heart failure entails polypharmacy, effective and rational. We employ polypharmacy in the treatment of chronic pain, and it can be effective, but it is not yet quite rational. Chronic pain is much too vague and uncertain an entity to allow us the luxury and convenience of treating it in a truly scientific manner. Therefore, our treatments are hit-or-miss, empiric, and symptom-directed. The tricyclics are helpful for pain and so are opiates, so we use both. SSRIs are helpful for depression, if not painfulness, so we use those also. The long-acting benzodiazepine, Klonopin, seems to help pain and certainly insomnia, so we add that. The short-acting benzodiazepine, Xanax, is good for anxiety, a common symptom of pain, so we add that too. The list goes on. Stimulants, anticonvulsants, and antipsychotics are all used in a glacially slow trial and error attempt to find the right combination of drugs.

No one, lay person or physician, looks askance at the use of three or four different drugs simultaneously for the treatment of diabetes, hypertension, cancer, arthritis, or heart disease. The use of an equal number of drugs for the treatment of chronic pain, however, invites suspicion. This is particularly so because the opiates, tranquilizers, stimulants, antidepressants, and anticonvulsants are all fatuously identified as *mind-altering drugs*. The belief that there are certain groups of drugs which are mind-altering is a thoughtless invention. Nearly all the drugs that we use today in clinical medicine, even including those for high blood pressure, arthritis, and control of heart rhythm, carry the potential to alter the mind.

Until we understand the biochemistry of pain, we will have to rely on clinical observation and our imagination.

There is a high degree of understanding about how drugs used in the treatment of diabetes and heart failure actually work. The degree of understanding about how mind-soul drugs work is, however, much less certain. We do know, at least at a primitive level, why an anticonvulsant works for epilepsy, a stimulant for attention deficit disorder, an antipsychotic for schizophrenia, and an antidepressant for that disease. We don't begin to understand, really, why so many of them work for pain. It is a profound enigma, and the answer will almost certainly not be discovered for decades. Until we understand the biochemistry of pain, we will have to rely on clinical observation and our imagination.

There are but few things we really know about chronic pain. We know that it begins with antecedents of remarkable variety, many of them psychiatric disorders. It is associated with behavioral effects, vast in number, but somewhat predictable. And it responds to many drugs with many different pharmacologic properties. These observations are true and above challenge by anyone. How do we make sense of it? Only, I believe, by exploring the fascinating interplay of chronic pain and disorders of the mind. The different forms of chronic pain overlap and merge with one another in their clinical display. Psychiatric disorders also merge with each other. Depression, mania, substance abuse, insomnia, conversion, obsessions, and delusions are all interrelated. Many patients experience several of these throughout the course of their lives, just as patients with chronic pain experience many different painful diseases throughout their lives.

CHAPTER SIX

Memory

The experience of pain cannot be separated, as we shall see time and time again, from the experiences of sleep, appetite, thought, mood, and memory. Let's explore the act of memory and its role in the generation of illness, painful and otherwise.

A life event, sufficient in meaning to command attention, invokes a change within the brain. Neurons dedicated to the acquisition of memory are recruited (the brain has enormous reserves of cells for this purpose) and they undergo a transformation. The arrangement of their neurotransmitters and receptors is altered in response to a new and previously unlearned experience. This process takes time, perhaps as long as a few minutes. As we all know, the act of rote memorization takes a while, and as we also know, a recently acquired memory is one of the most fragile things in nature, easily lost by distraction or the diversion of attention to other matters. Given sufficient time, however, the act of memorization is completed, and an experience is stored away, forever available for recall.

Kindred memories are stored by kindred cells. There is a brain-place for remembered words, another for remembered music, and almost certainly another for remembered pain. Memories are acquired along the dimension of time, and they are layered that way, one on top of the other. The most remote experiences are ensconced together, deep within the brain substance, and the more recently acquired, sequentially on top. The recall of a memory will therefore often invoke other temporally associated memories. For example, a listener hearing a remembered tune may recall the occasion of its first hearing. He may remember the theater, the companion of the evening, the dinner before the performance, and perhaps even the vintage of wine selected for the occasion. The association of memories within brain-place and brain-time can be operative, as we shall see shortly, in the generation of very complex diseases.

We usually think of memory as an *experiential* phenomenon. It is a product of consciousness. We experience something that commands our awareness, and we register it as memory. A memory, however, is nothing more than a rearrangement of neurotransmitters on the surface of the neuron. This rearrangement may be induced, as we shall also see, by the introduction of certain chemicals into the brain. These agents incite a change in the neurotransmitter configuration that will last forever. They create a sort of biologic memory beyond any recall to consciousness, but available nonetheless to reappear when circumstances warrant.

There is another form of biologic memory that is induced not by chemicals but by alien living organisms. Chicken pox is a common disease of childhood. It is usually a rather trivial and unmemorable illness (few of us actually recall the experience). The body's defenses overwhelm but do not quite destroy the virus. It retreats and finds domicile within that portion of the neural architecture known as the dorsal root ganglion. The ganglia (there are several of them) are arranged segmentally along the spinal cord. They house the sensory nerves. Filaments (axons) from these extend out to the skin where they are stimulated by touch, heat, cold, or pain. Their excitation sends a message to the ganglion where it is relayed up into the brain for interpretation. For some reason, only God knows why, the chicken pox virus is able to continue living only within the ganglion. It exists there as a sort of biologic memory, beyond any measure of conscious control, but capable of resurrection when invited to do so. The administration of drugs, such as cortisone, which diminish immunologic competence, may restore the virus to activity. Intercurrent illness and emotional stress may also do it. The virus suddenly springs into vigor, replicates, and spreads. It follows the path of least resistance, infiltrating and inflaming the nerve axon all the way out to the skin. This produces the disease we know as herpes zoster, or shingles.

The migraineur possesses an arrangement of cells and their neurotransmitters which are dedicated, again only God knows why, to the generation of headache. In most cases this arrangement is dictated by genetics, but sometimes by infection or head trauma. Regardless of its origin, it is, in a true sense, a form of biologic memory. The migraine headache is a remembered behavior. Like all memories, it is subject to resurrection when circumstances (triggers) dictate.

Harry was an estimable man—he was tall, erect, gray, intelligent, and well-spoken—a serious person. We were introduced by a mutual friend, a psychiatrist. Harry was having trouble swallowing. Food seemed to hang up in his gullet, and he had a sense of fullness and pressure in his chest, and he was losing weight. X-rays confirmed Harry had cancer of the esophagus. It extended through the esophageal wall into the lymph nodes of the chest. It was beyond surgical resection. I treated him with radiotherapy hoping for a few months of palliation. During his treatment I got to know him well. He had been alcoholic in his youth. In his mid-twenties, he entered recovery under the aegis of Alcoholics Anonymous. He became a member of that organization and a Presbyterian minister. He had many friends and callers. They came in number to sit by his bedside.

Cancer of the esophagus occurs with high frequency in alcoholics. We can surmise that the exposure of the mucosal surface to the cytotoxic chemical, ethyl alcohol, incites within these cells a chromosomal aberration. Harry had not used alcohol for many years, even decades, and yet, we can be sure, the rules still apply. His alcoholism was almost certainly the cause of his esophageal cancer. His exposure to the drug began in his teens when highly plastic cells were proliferating in organizational development. The cells of the esophagus suffered an injury resulting in a chromosomal reconfiguration. The abnormal cells were recognized as alien by immunosurveillance, and they were suppressed and inhibited, but not destroyed. Like the chicken pox virus, they remained viable, a form of biologic memory subject to reappearance. With advancing age and diminishing immunologic competence, they found expression as carcinoma of the esophagus. The knowledgeable reader will immediately recognize that there is quite a difference between an acquired chromosomal reconfiguration and an acquired neuronal transmitter reconfiguration. One leads to cancer. The other does not. Both, however, constitute a memory, capable of finding expression years removed.

Harry's cancer reappeared, and I admitted him to the hospital for terminal care. He was weakened but alert. He remained ever gracious and civil until he developed, over the course of a day or two, a change in his behavior. His pulse and blood pressure rose, and he became more restless. These developments were not entirely unexpected. Anxiety, confusion, and restlessness are common in terminal illness. In Harry's case, however, it went beyond that. He rapidly evolved into a raging delirium. He became agitated and tremulous and experienced fearful hallucination of strange creatures in his room and in his bed. Harry had developed delirium tremens.

The disease in its fullest expression is easily recognizable, but rare is the physician who identifies it as it first develops. It always seems to sneak up on us. It certainly did with me, and with cause. Harry had not had a drink for many years, and delirium tremens occurs, by definition, within a finite time following the cessation of alcohol, a few days to a couple of weeks at the most. Harry didn't fulfill the diagnostic criteria for delirium tremens. We have another name for Harry's condition—alcoholic hallucinosis. But it is the same disease; we just employ different semantics.

My psychiatrist friend, more knowledgeable in these matters than I, recognized the problem immediately and told me, "I know it has been years since he has had a drink of alcohol, but that is still an alcoholic brain. Give him some Valium." Harry calmed down in a short while. He became again a sentient being and a few days later died quietly and with dignity, appropriate to his illustrious life.

To digress a bit, I had a treatment choice with Harry. He suffered delirium, a form of psychosis. His thought was disordered. He saw things that were not there. It probably related to some uninhibited release of dopamine in critical brain cells. I could have treated him, as we used to do, with antipsychotic drugs. These are dopamine-blocking agents, and they would have worked, but they would have worked slowly. Again, most drugs which alter the sero-tonin, noradrenaline, and dopamine axis require an interval of days or weeks before they become operative. This is their hallmark. For this reason, they are poor drugs for the treatment of delirium tremens which is a life-threatening disorder, one needful of a quick-acting drug. Valium requires no neuronal reconfiguration for its effect. It immediately enhances the release of gamma-aminobutyric acid, the brain's inhibitory or calming neurotransmitter.

Harry's brain, in its plastic, developmental youth, had acquired, by virtue of repeated exposure to a false neurotransmitter, ethyl alcohol, a reconfiguration which required for its effective func-tioning the presence of that neurotransmitter. When Harry entered recovery, this system was rendered inoperative and unneeded, but remained extant and subject to reappearance if circumstance invited. In Harry's case it was a visceral cancer. A latent neural configuration, a biologic memory, one dependent upon the pres-ence of ethyl alcohol for its function, became operative and, starved for that neurotransmitter, found an expression in an illness, delirium tremens. I could have treated Harry with intravenous alcohol. It would have worked quite well, but he would have to die a few days later inebriated. Hardly a worthy end. Valium is better.

Odell served in Europe in World War II and saw sustained action in the Battle of the Bulge. I asked him several times to tell me about it, but his responses were always guarded and hesitant. I ascribed this to his innate reserve, unaware of the real reason. Unable or unwilling to tell me of his experiences, Odell did invite me to read about them. He brought me his diary of his months in Europe. Each day's events, whether trivial or grand, were entered without elaboration or reflection. The great battle and the loss of comrades were recorded with no comment on the meaning of the events. There was no sense of sadness or pride in his or his unit's achievements other than the singular notation that his weapon fired more rounds in one day in the Battle of the Bulge than the Long Tom Howitzer had ever fired before.

When I returned the diary and offered my appreciation, Odell lost his reserve. His eyes lit up, and he became expansive. "We hurt them, Doc. We hurt them real bad. I saw it. Our guns killed a lot of Germans. Yesiree, a lot of Germans." And then he hesitated. He choked and flushed. His eyes moistened, and he abruptly left the room without a word of goodbye to me or my staff. I resolved never to bring the subject up again.

A few weeks later my nurse led me into my office, closed the door, and said, "You have to take this call. I can't handle it. Odell just tried to kill his wife." She had spoken something hurtful, and Odell exploded. He doused her with paint thinner and slammed the truck door on her legs. He told her that if she ever crossed him again he would kill her. The children had taken her to their home to sequester her, and then called me for advice. There were the usual strictures. The police were not to be called, and I was called only in great confidentiality. "Don't dare tell Odell we told you about this. He will kill us all."

A few days later he appeared in my office, phlegmatic and slow as always. It was time for his cholesterol check. I broke a confidence and told him that I had heard some terrible things. "She just crossed me, Doc. Lots of things cross me now. Even the people in church bother me. I didn't use to be that way."

A sweet man had experienced a total change in his behavior. Was it the irascibility of an approaching senility? Was it a psychosis, a derangement of thought? Or alcohol? Or an agitated depression? I proceeded gently with my inquiry and began by asking him about his sleep. I always do because disordered sleep is an important clue to emotional disintegration. Odell offered an elaborate lie. "It's strange, Doc. You know I have a big prostate, and my bladder is active. It keeps me awake at night, but I finally figured out that if I stay up real late before I go to bed, I can go right to sleep. My bladder doesn't bother so much." Then he began to weep. After what seemed an interminable period of time, his speech returned and he said, "Doc, every night when I go to bed, I sleep with dead Germans."

A memory, a horrific memory, the carnage of the battlefield— repressed and sequestered for fifty years, but recrudescing as an expression of depressive illness. Odell's disease was probably multifactorial. He was well into his seventies and beginning to experience some cognitive decline with loss of control. He certainly had entered a major depression, potentially destructive to himself and others. He also suffered post-traumatic stress disorder with flashbacks to a dreadful experience. A terrible event was endured, then incorporated and sequestered into memory, subject to reappearance in a disease state characterized by disordered sleep and depression.

Our memories, good and bad, are housed within our cerebral apparatus, each within a nidus of cells whose interplay has been facilitated by remote events. They lie there, unused but available for recall to consciousness when circumstance commands. Odell's circumstance was depression. The workings of his brain entered a new configuraton, and by doing so, facilitated the expression of unpleasant memoires. Odell's flashbacks occurred during sleep, which, as most of us surely know, is also a potent activator of memory in the form of dreams. Depression and sleep are also provocateurs of biologic memories. Migraine often worsens during depression and, in some people, headache occurs only at night.

Dean suffered a compression fracture of a thoracic vertebrae. It was an uncomplicated fracture. There was no damage to his spinal cord and nerve roots, but as is typical with the disorder, he suffered pain for several weeks. He ultimately recovered as his fracture stabilized, and he entered a state of wellness. But, we can be sure, his painful experience was imprinted in his neural matrix as memory. A segment of his brain had acquired a back-is-hurting configuration, and that configuration was operative for an interval of several weeks. Then, unnecessary and unwanted, it was stored away. An experiential memory had become a biologic memory subject, as they all are, to resurrection. Years later, when he developed coronary artery disease, he experienced the pain of his myocardial ischemia not in his chest or his arm or his jaw, but only in his mid-back, precisely at the site of his remote fracture. A painful memory, latent but convenient and available, was recruited years later into clinical expression by a new and unrelated disease.

The recruitment of an old pain by a new pain may seem strange and bizarre and might be dismissed by many readers as mere coincidence. It is not. It happens all the time. We have only to look at migraine. The migraineur has a highly developed neural configuration dedicated to the creation of headache. This complex system, fully arrayed, ready, and responsive is recruited by a number of triggers. Among these, and this is probably not widely appreciated, is the occurrence of pain in the head or face. A neck sprain, a concussion, or an infected tooth can all precipitate migraine. They do this simply by presenting to the brain a painful signal which excites a remembered and readily available behavior, that of migraine. It happens all the time.

Michelle was involved in an automobile accident, a minor fender-bender. Her car was struck from the rear, and her neck hyperextended. She suffered a whiplash injury, and within a short while began experiencing neck stiffness and pain radiating from her shoulder down through her left arm into her middle finger. This was a typical scenario for a ruptured cervical disc, but her MRI studies and electromyogram were normal. Her physical examination showed a full range of motion in the neck and shoulder and normal sensation, strength, and reflexes. It also showed the scar of a gunshot wound beneath her left collarbone, a feature that certainly demanded attention. Some three years before, while working at a convenience store, she was robbed at gun point and then shot through the left upper chest, the bullet passing through the network of neural trunks known as the brachial plexus. She suffered a nerve injury, immediately experiencing pain in the arm, hand, and left middle finger. Her pain continued for several weeks and then gradually dissipated. She had experienced a nerve contusion which, with time, (neural injuries are notoriously slow to heal) resolved. Then three years later, a car wreck had provoked an identical painful syndrome. With no other obvious accountant for her pain, such as a ruptured disc, it was reasonable to conclude that a remotely damaged and scarred nerve was rendered susceptible to further injury, in this case by a stretch due to neck hyperextension. Her pain was a memory of sort, but a very primitive memory—a simple mechanical disfigurement of the nerve. I could reasonably expect her gradual recovery, much as happened the first time, but, weeks into her illness, Michelle was not improving. She was getting worse. Her sleep was interrupted by nightmares, and she was fatigued, depressed, and losing weight. Why these effects, appearing and getting worse, as she should have been getting better? As is almost always the case in the painful patient, there was something else going on. All it took was a little asking.

After her gunshot wound, Michelle suffered nightmares and flashbacks to her assailant and her wounding. Her physician recognized her post-traumatic stress disorder and treated her with Valium. Her flashbacks, insomnia, and anxiety went away gradually, as did her arm pain. She discarded her Valium and got on with her life, at least until her automobile accident. Immediately following that event, as her left arm pain developed, she experienced, you guessed it, the reappearance of flashbacks to her assailant and her wounding. A remote experiential memory was recruited by a minor stressor, a fender-bender. What then, was the genesis of her pain? Was it simply the exacerbation of a remote neural injury? Was her post-traumatic stress disorder simply an add-on, totally unrelated to her pain? Hardly. The two should not and cannot be separated. Her clinical course, her failure to recover, suggested that something was amiss, that there was more than just nerve injury. The concurrence of her stress disorder with her pain opened the door for me (there is almost always a door available for the painful patient if you look hard enough). I knew, at the least, that she would not get better until I treated her stress disorder. That done, I could hope for one of two scenarios—the slow resolution of her pain as her injured nerve regenerated at its glacial pace or, if we were lucky, pretty rapid improvement in her pain allowing a couple of weeks for the drugs to kick in. That is exactly what happened. I gave her the tricyclic Imipramine and the benzodiazepine Klonopin. Her flashbacks and anxiety dissipated, and her pain was gone—totally gone—within a short while.

Michelle's pain was segmental, inclusive to the seventh cervical nerve. Such pain by all rights should originate in that nerve and not in the brain. Neural architecture within the brain does not reflect the function of a single peripheral nerve. There has been too much admixture and intermingling for that. It is unlikely that a brain lesion could produce pain solely in the distribution of the seventh cervical nerve. Quite unlikely, that is, unless we incorporate the phenomenon of memory. Just as there are brain cells dedicated to the memory of dead Germans or the memory of back pain, there was in Michelle a group of cells dedicated to the memory of a brachial plexus injury. And those cells, it takes no leap of faith here, were in her closely assimilated with another memory, that of assault. Just accept for a while that it could happen this way. It is the only way we are going to understand painfulness.

CHAPTER SEVEN

Triavil

Margaret was in her seventies, a graceful and beautiful person, but suffering head pain. Several years before she had experienced attacks of recurrent, brief, lancinating pains about her right eye. Tic douloureux (trigeminal neuralgia) occurs typically in midlife or later, and it has many causes, but it is often due to pressure on the Gasserian ganglion by a dilated and tortuous carotid artery. The Gasserian is like the dorsal root ganglion, only much larger. It houses the cells which receive sensation from the richly enervated face and head. Its irritation by a pounding artery could certainly be expected to produce pain. An operation to displace the artery away from the ganglion by placing a pledget between them was performed, and Margaret obtained relief from her tic pain. Then, years later, she developed recurrent pain, something like a tic, but not quite. Her pain was confined to the right upper face, but was more widespread and diffuse than before and much longer in duration, lasting an hour or even more. It recurred three or four times daily. It was hard to delineate with certainty the nature of her pain. It was clearly related in some manner to her prior tic, encompassing the same approximate anatomic area, but its duration was too long for a typical tic pain. In its repetitiveness and stereotyped nature, it was somewhat like migraine, but the recurrence, up to several times daily, was unusual even for that disorder. Such frequency of recurrence does occur in that migraine variant known as cluster headaches, but that is a disease of middle-aged males and not elderly females. It is also a disease associated with certain stigmata that make it rather easy to identify. Margaret had none of these. She did not have cluster headaches. She did, however, have a remote history of very typical migraine. Her headaches lasted a day or two and occurred randomly through the course of her life but abated, as migraine often does, when she entered her maturity. Margaret's face pain, I suspected, represented a hybrid of two different pain syndromes. It lasted too long for a tic, but was too short for a migraine. It had something of both. It was an incorporation of two separate painful memories, a melding of tic and migraine. This merging of pain syndromes, quite different in their etiology, but located in proximate areas of the body, is by no means uncommon. This should not surprise. Our memory is, after all, imperfect.

As Margaret had become painful she had also become depressed. Painfulness and depression frequently occur together. In her case, however, there may have been special meaning. Years before, when she was in her forties, she suffered a depression severe enough to require electroconvulsive therapy. I suspected that her depression represented the recrudescence of a remembered behavior. I was rather sure her face pain did.

I had an interesting choice of treatments, an SSRI or a tricyclic for depression and Sansert or Depakote for migraine, or even Tegretol (well-established in the treatment of tic). Any or all of these would have been reasonable therapy, and I tried most of them but with limited success. As I went along trying this and that drug, my history taking offered me a new insight. During her depression, she had been treated with Triavil, and had remained on that drug for several years.

Triavil is little used now and may not be known to many readers, but it is a remarkable drug, one of the really great drugs of recent medical history. It is a combination of two agents, Trilafon, an antipsychotic, dopamine-blocking agent, and Amitriptyline, a tricyclic. It came out about thirty-five years ago for the treatment of depression, anxiety, and insomnia. It is quite evident now, but was less so then, that it was too much drug for what it was intended. Most of the newer pharmaceuticals are highly specific for a single neurotransmitter, often a single neurotransmitter subtype. This specificity is desirable. It gives us a cleaner drug and one, hopefully, with fewer side effects. Triavil has no such specificity. It affects multiple neurotransmitter systems. The metabolism of serotonin, noradrenaline, and dopamine are all altered by its persuasion. We never had before, nor in the future will have, a single pill as multiply active and omnipotent as Triavil. Among all the drugs we have ever used for the treatment of mind disease, Triavil is nonpareil. It insinuates itself into the totality

The brain is a complex place, and it may exhibit a variety of responses to drug therapy.

of the cerebral machinery to an extent unequaled, for good or bad, by any other drug. The combination of an antipsychotic and an antidepressant for the treatment of anxiety and simple insomnia is, in retrospect, unseemly. At the time, however, Triavil was a very attractive drug for one very good reason. It was non-addictive, and the drugs it was competing with, Meprobamate and later Valium, certainly were. For that reason we welcomed and used the heavy-handed Triavil, and it was remarkably effective, it seemed for almost everything. Depression, anxiety, insomnia, migraine, irritable bowels, and even schizophrenia all responded. For an interval of a few decades, Triavil was one of the most prescribed psychiatric drugs. Then it fell into eclipse. Many patients on the drug, over extended periods of time, developed the syndrome of tardive dyskinesia. This is a movement disorder, not dissimilar to dystonia. It consists of repetitive lip-smacking and grimacing facial movements. It was due, we can be sure, to the effects of long-term dopamine blockade. Triavil, formerly so helpful, became almost overnight a bad and dangerous drug. It also became a cottage industry, employing hundreds of lawyers around the country as they pursued litigation.

Physicians abandoned Triavil, but in some cases it was hard to do. Many patients would not tolerate abstinence from the drug. Triavil is not a true addictive agent, but as a combination of chemicals that incorporate themselves into the totality of the cerebral apparatus, it does leave a legacy. Cessation of the drug occasionally produced a type of withdrawal with nausea, tremulousness, and restlessness. In other cases it would produce extravagant recurrence of depression, migraine, or schizophrenia. Astonishingly, cessation of the drug would occasionally produce tardive dyskinesia! Amazing stuff. Long-term exposure to Triavil caused tardive dyskinesia in some patients, and in others cessation of the drug caused the same disorder. Too much of the drug and not enough of the drug did the same thing. Incredible? Not really. The brain is a complex place, and it may exhibit a variety of responses to drug therapy.

Margaret was depressed, and she suffered head pain that could not be clearly identified as either migraine or tic douloureux. I tried all the right drugs but without success. Then, when all else failed, I prescribed Triavil. I knew that the drug always seemed to work best in the patient who didn't quite fit, who was on the edge of the diagnostic tables. I also knew that Triavil was a drug that left its mark. Sometimes the reinstitution of Triavil was the only effective way to treat depression or migraine. Margaret's depression ameliorated, her sleep returned, and her face pain went away.

Triavil can be, even in this era, an appropriate therapeutic agent. It was in Margaret. She had suffered tic doloureaux, migraine, and depression on separate occasions through her life. These experiential and behavioral memories were sequestered in her neural matrix and reappeared, albeit in the form of a hybrid, in her maturity. The hybrid was unresponsive to conventional therapy. It responded, however, very well to Triavil. The remembered experience of painfulness and depression, however modified, was treated successfully by the incorporation of a remembered pharmacy.

Lucy was in her late thirties, lean and athletic. She was hiking with companions through the Smokies, lost her footing, fell, and rolled for a short way down a ledge. She was banged up a bit, but there were no major injuries. She climbed back up to the trail and concluded her hike inconvenienced only slightly by discomfort in her shoulders and back. The next day there was more muscular soreness and stiffness. She took over-the-counter analgesics and anticipated her recovery in a few days, but it didn't happen. As the weeks passed her pain worsened, spreading to her neck, low back, and buttocks. She became sleepless, and attempts to sleep were disturbed by muscle jerkings and restless legs. She consulted her physician and was given a muscle relaxant, but she did not respond. She then began, as so many painful patients do, her journey among the consultants—orthopedists, neurologists, and neurosurgeons. Her tests, MRIs, myelograms, and electromyograms were all normal. Physical therapy was initiated, but as is sometimes the case, it was extraordinarily painful to her. She began to gain weight, and she became depressed. She had developed fibromyalgia, seemingly initiated by a minor muscular injury. She had failed to recover.

When I first saw her it seemed that she was really no different from other patients with fibromyalgia, although her pain behaviors and her evident distress were remarkable. I gave her in sequence several different tricyclics and benzodiazepines, but the effects were marginal at best. This was unusual. The drugs are a long way from perfect, but in nearly everyone they provide at least some relief. This was not the case with Lucy. She was going to be different, I could tell that.

There were a number of trigger points in her back and neck, and these were very sensitive. Palpation would produce extravagant pain. She would cry out and grimace when these were touched, even lightly. Her movements were hesitant and protective. Lying on the examining table was a stressful act, accompanied by grunting and shifting about to find a comfortable posture. Her gait was affected. She kept her hand against the wall as she walked, and she would lean on any available object to help support her weight. As time went by and my attempts at treatment failed, I knew I was seeing something very unusual. Her behaviors were exaggerated to an extent I had never seen before.

I was not then and am not now enamored of that form of treatment known as trigger point injections. The painful areas are identified and injected with cortisone and a local anesthetic, followed by massage, this in an effort to break up the localized painful muscle spasm. It is not a very graceful form of treatment, but I was getting nowhere with my drugs, so I referred Lucy to the anesthesiologist for trigger point injections. It didn't go well at all. She screamed with pain with each injection and thrashed about the bed in agony. The procedures were terminated, but Lucy's violent pain behaviors continued.

Burns, heart attacks, and kidney stones can produce terrible pains but even in the worst cases, the victim remains a sentient being, able to respond and at least attempt to obey commands. Not so with Lucy. She was insensate to every stimulus except her pain. She could not respond or obey. She could only writhe in bed and scream. There was no indication of visceral damage. No needle-too-deep lung injury, a pneumothorax. Her blood oxygenation was good, and her cardiographic monitor showed no evidence of myocardial injury, only a sustained tachycardia, hardly unexpected in this setting. She was sweaty and clammy, and her pupils were dilated to an extent that the iris was hardly evident. I gave her intravenous morphine, and she quickly calmed down. She fell asleep, and her pulse and blood pressure stabilized. After her nap she was able to move about again, hesitantly, but at least reactive and appropriate. I called a friend to drive her home, instructing her to have Lucy return to see me in a few days.

She was, for her, calm and stable when she came back. She professed no resentment at our misadventure, but she remained, as before, stooped, limping, and posturing to protect herself from pain. She and I talked about the experience which, in my naïveté and perhaps my bias, I judged to be exaggerated and perhaps even histrionic (hysteric). I requested a referral to a psychiatrist. She acquiesced. "I don't think it will help, but I will try it if it will make me better."

I had resolved at this juncture that this patient, whose behaviors and reactions to her pain were so amplified, suffered some form of personality disorder. Personality disorders exist in many forms, paranoid, histrionic, passive-dependent, and others. They represent ingrained and lifelong maladaptive behaviors characterized, most of them, by some degree of anxiety and a just-don't-get-it-quite-right pattern of existence. An intercurrent illness in a patient with a personality disorder can be a very destructive experience. I was sure this would be the explanation in Lucy. I welcomed the psychiatrist's opinion.

I had, of course, in my frustration come to blame the patient for her disease. She had not responded to my very appropriate treatments. There just had to be something in her psychologic makeup to cause her to behave so strangely. I failed to note, however, that Lucy, before her illness, was an effective, gainfully employed, and reasonably content individual whose life, it seemed, had in no way been marked by any kind of behavioral disturbance.

I received the psychiatrist's judgment a few days later. Depression due to chronic pain. No evidence of any kind of personality disorder. I had reached the end of the line with Lucy. I had tried and tried hard to find that form of treatment which would make some inroads on her disease, but I had failed abysmally. I suggested referral to another physician, but she declined. We separated, she to go her painful way, and I to mine, trying to forget this unfortunate experience as I treated other, more responsive patients.

It was several months later when Lucy showed up again, still painful, sleepless, and depressed. I was happy to see her, happy to get a second chance. After all, I had learned a lot since I last saw her. Maybe, somewhere, there was another door to open. Lucy told me, "You are a very good doctor. You tried to help me, and I appreciate it. I want you to try again." Quite a compliment, I thought, and I accepted it as such, but I realize now I shouldn't have. It was just a little too ingratiating, and I should have been on my guard. Fortunately things turned out pretty well for a while, but it could have been bad. Lucy later confided to me that she had not returned to get well. She had returned simply to obtain a supply of drugs sufficient to allow her to commit suicide.

I started over with Lucy, from the beginning. I recorded her history of wellness before her fall, her absolute failure to respond to what in sum amounted to a dozen or so different drugs, her remarkable painful behaviors, and her astonishing intolerance to trigger point injections and physical therapy. Armed with better knowledge and more experience, I inquired if she had ever taken the drug Triavil. Yes, she replied. She remembered it. She had taken it as a teenager for several years for her migraine headaches. Triavil in a teenager! The most potent neuropsychiatric drug ever, introduced into the plastic brain of a child.

We are beginning to understand that throughout life our brains are creating new neurons. This act, we can be sure, occurs not willy-nilly, but in response to a stimulus. Could the administration of a drug which alters a host of neurotransmitter actions be such a stimulus? Is it possible that the introduction of a drug invokes the creation of cells dedicated to its effect on neurotransmission? Beyond possible, it is even likely.

Is it possible that the introduction of a drug invokes the creation of cells dedicated to its effect on neurotransmission? Beyond possible, it is even likely.

I was about to perform a delicious clinical experiment, but I didn't tell Lucy it was an experiment. I told her that there was great likelihood that the readministration of Triavil would help her, perhaps a lot. I felt sure that it would, and there was no holding back. I employed every power of suggestion and positive reinforcement I could. I was playing my last card. I was hopeful, really hopeful, and she sensed it. I gave her a prescription for a hundred pills, a quantity sufficient for a successful suicide, but I directed her, at least initially, to take only one pill each night.

She called the next morning to report that she slept well and was already less stiff and sore than she had been in two years. I repeated instructions to slowly increase the dosage to three pills nightly and to see me again in a couple of weeks. Triavil is slow in onset of action. Its clinical effect usually requires several days. The neuronal reconfiguration again. It takes time. But in Lucy it took only a little. Her improvement was almost immediate. Overnight she felt better. Why? It is hard to say for certain, but there is a reasonable working hypothesis. Her cerebral machinery, including her analgesic system (remember, she had been given the drug for a painful disease—migraine) had been rearranged by exposure to Triavil. With her fall, this system came under the provocation of a painful signal. Her cerebral apparatus was starved for Triavil in the same manner that the patient with delirium tremens is starved for alcohol. The response to reintroduction of the drug was immediate. No reorganization was required.

She was a happy camper when I saw her next, ebullient and charming. I liked her a lot and was ashamed that I had misdiagnosed her painful behavior as the product of personality disorder. I should have known better. Lucy did well—for a while. I made minor adjustments in her dosages, manipulating the relative quantities of her drugs. She gained a lot of weight, as Triavil-treated patients often do, but she expressed no remorse. "I don't mind being fat. At last I am free of pain." It went nicely for a good while, several months, and Lucy and I enjoyed our visits. Then the wheels came off. She experienced the phenomenon of *tachyphylaxis*, that is, the drug simply quit working. She became gradually more painful and sleepless in spite of ever higher dosage, and in the last happy move I made in her treatment, I added Lithium. Once again she got better and remained so for several months, but then her disease recurred inexorably. I pushed drug doses to the maximum, but with each incremental increase there was only slight benefit. After a year or so of wellness, she relapsed totally into destructive painfulness and left me again, this time to seek solace in opiates purchased on the streets and through forged prescriptions. Remarkably, she also forged prescriptions for Triavil. She continued to take the drug in ever increasing amounts. More and more of it. Always bigger doses to get just a little more relief.

I saw her several weeks later in the emergency room. She was comatose, and her heart and respiratory rates accelerated. Chest x-rays showed a pulmonary edema pattern and the electrocardio-gram the telltale widening of electrical complexes due to tricyclic drug intoxication. Her Amitriptyline level was at potentially lethal heights. I admitted her into the intensive care unit and pulled in my resources, cardiologists and pulmonologists. She never required ventilator support. Watchful waiting and the passage of time seemed to be in order. I gave her diuretics to improve her pulmonary edema, but they didn't work very well. She did not have pulmonary edema imposed by fluid overload as occurs with congestive heart failure. Hers was a form of *neurogenic* pulmonary edema. In some circumstances, notably head injury and drug intox-ication, the capillary vessels of the lungs become inflamed and permeable, and the pulmonary air spaces fill with fluid. There is no specific treatment, only support.

As Lucy regained consciousness over a few days and recounted the story of her drug usage, I pleaded with her that she go to a treatment center for withdrawal from her opiates. She refused. She was sure that her pain would only worsen. She accepted discharge from the hospital with appreciation for my effort, but with no desire to return to my care.

I don't know where Lucy is now. I hope she is all right, but I doubt it. I have a pretty good idea about how it all ended up. She did teach me so much. No conclusions here, only speculation, but I wonder if her painful disease was generated by prior exposure to Triavil. Would she have developed her relentless painfulness had she not received the drug as a child? We will never know, but I kind of doubt it.

Harriet, in her sixties, experienced a series of small strokes. Her speech and her cognition were impaired. She became anxious, sleepless, and depressed, not unexpected behaviors at all in this setting. I treated her with Triavil. The use of an antidepressant combined with an antipsychotic in a brain-damaged depressed patient was very reasonable therapy. She recovered from her depression completely, and nearly so from her strokes. She discontinued her Triavil therapy.

Several years later she developed a very queer illness. She became sleepless and abdomen-painful. Her pain was feeding-dependent. The ingestion of food was followed by a burning sensation in her gullet that coursed through her abdomen into her rectum. She avoided food and rapidly lost weight. There was no nausea or vomiting or change in bowel function. She evidenced no depression or anxiety. She was her usual upbeat self except that she was painful, losing weight rapidly, and quite unable to sleep.

A visceral malignancy was suspect although a rather unlikely accountant for the bizarre distribution of her pain or for that matter her sleeplessness. Her blood tests were in order. A CAT scan of the chest and abdomen was performed and revealed no

evidence of cancer, but it did show, surprisingly, a pericardial effusion, an accumulation of fluid around the heart. I referred her to a
cardiologist for his evaluation. He confirmed the presence of a
pericardial effusion, but recorded that her cardiac function otherwise was quite good. Harriet had pericarditis, but as is not
infrequently the case, the etiology was uncertain. Her fluid accumulation was significant but not critical, and she had no
complaints relative to her heart or lungs. Her pericardial disease
was quite asymptomatic. As best we could tell, it had no bearing
on her abdominal pain and sleeplessness. The cardiologist
concluded that watchful waiting was in order. He instructed her to
call him if she developed shortness of breath or chest pain and to
return for re-evaluation in a month.

Harriett came back to me, and I continued my investigation by
referring her to a gastroenterologist to see if he could determine by
endoscopy the cause of her abdominal pain and weight loss. It was
unremarkable. There was no evidence of disease in her stomach,
colon, or small bowel. The gastroenterologist signed off. She
returned for my disposition, and I treated her with Triavil. I knew
that Triavil seemed to work best in those patients whose symptoms
didn't fit in any certain diagnostic category, and I knew she had
received it before with benefit. I anticipated that it would help.

Harriet was exhibiting, as many patients do, the appearance of
her disease in fragments and partials. Neuropsychiatric illnesses, at
least at their onset, rarely appear as discrete, full-blown, recognizable entities. Arrayed over a scale of time, they appear piecemeal
and gradually. I felt that her painfulness, weight loss, and insomnia
represented a *forme fruste*, an incomplete expression of a recurrent
depression. Her pericarditis, I supposed, was an unrelated issue, and
I left that problem in the hands of the cardiologist.

She responded immediately to Triavil. Sleep was restored. Her
painfulness abated. Her appetite returned, and she began to gain
weight. Cardiac sonography done a short while later showed no
evidence of pericardial effusion. The cardiologist sent me a note.
He was happy that she had recovered, but was, even in retrospect,
unable to account for her disease.

Let's ask an interesting question. Did Harriet's pericarditis respond to Triavil? At first pass, it seems unlikely. Few cardiologists would remotely accept that possibility. It is almost too whimsical to merit serious consideration, but let's look at the other side of the coin. If her pericardial disease was unrelated to her behavioral and painful disease, she had then experienced simultaneously two separate and unrelated illnesses, one functional and the other organic and had, in a remarkable display of coincidence, been cured of both at virtually the same time. Not a very likely scenario at all.

The heart, lungs, and viscera are subject to neural control. No one would contest this. Cardiovascular functions are profoundly altered by emotional circumstance and mood. They are also altered by head injury and drug intoxication. These, we know with certainty, can cause neurogenic pulmonary edema. Could there not be neurogenic pericarditis? Could neural dysfunction in the form of disordered mood or medication effect actually inflame the pericardium? I believe it can, and I suspect it happened in Harriet. Pulmonary edema and pericarditis are not dissimilar diseases. One is a disorder of the lining of blood vessels and the other of the lining of the heart. The search for a common etiology of both is by no means unwarranted. If we look, however, for a common causation generated by drug effects, we find a paradox. Lucy's pulmonary edema was due to too much Triavil. Harriet's pericarditis, it seems, was due to too little. Lucy's pulmonary edema went away when we stopped Triavil. Harriet's pericarditis when we started it! The paradox may not be all that it seems. Too much and too little don't mean quite the same in the brain as they do in the heart or the lungs. Remember tardive dyskinesia. It appears in some patients after they have been on Triavil too long, and in others when the drug is discontinued.

Lucy's pulmonary edema and Harriet's pericarditis were the result of the biologic phenomenon known as *neurogenic inflammation*. The capacity of disordered neural cells to produce an inflammatory reaction is widely recognized by neurologists, perhaps less by other physicians. It is thought to be an accountant for the remarkable variety of inflammatory events generated by migraine, be this stroke, nerve palsy, or swelling and hemorrhage into the scalp.

Neurogenic inflammation probably accounts for much more than migraine. More on this subject later.

Many psychiatrists, I am sure, have shared the experience of reintroducing Triavil therapy with benefit in depressed patients. Its utility in painful states in those previously exposed to the drug is perhaps less well-appreciated, but from the cases presented above, I doubt the effect can be seriously questioned. But the notion that Triavil might relieve a pericardial effusion is alien and suspect. This is principally, almost exclusively, because of our propensity to separate the mind from the body, and to disassemble them into separate compartments. The mind-body dichotomy. It does not exist. Behavior and biology are inseparable.

CHAPTER EIGHT

The Painful Brain

T he experience of pain, as I have suggested before, is kindred to
the experiences of thought and mood. They are housed in the
same brain-places and controlled by the same brain chemicals
(neurotransmitters). The other senses, those of vision, hearing, and
touch, are housed in very different brain-places and controlled by
different transmitters. Pain, therefore, is unique among the senses.
Only occasionally do sight and sound provoke emotional and
behavioral reactions. Pain *always* does.

It is time to pause and discuss, briefly, the manner in which our
brains work. This is the necessary groundwork for understanding
the case histories that follow. We actually have two brains. They are
interactive, interdependent, and mutually supportive, but they are
in a very real sense two separate organs. Our predominant brain, at
least in size, is the cerebral cortex. The gray matter on the surface,
it constitutes some 90 percent of the total brain's cellular volume. It
employs in its operations two major neurotransmitters, glutamic
acid, which is excitatory, and gamma-aminobutyric acid, which is
inhibitory. Cortical neurons are vastly complicated in their aggregate, but individually they are rather simple mechanisms. They
function as stop-go systems. Glutamic acid is go. GABA is stop.
They are hard-wired and predictable in their function. The cortical
activities of movement, vision, audition, and tactile (touch) sensation are pretty much constant. They don't change from day to day.

The cerebral cortex is divided by a cleft into left and right
hemispheres. Each of these is further segmented into major lobes,
the occipital dedicated to the function of vision, the parietal to the

function of tactile sensation, the temporal to audition, and the frontal to motor function. It is a lateralized brain with each hemisphere subserving the perception of sensation and the control of movement in the opposite side of the body. Lateralization extends also into the faculty of speech and motor dominance, in most of us in the left hemisphere. The cortical brain is highly topographic. Specific areas of each lobe are dedicated to specific functions, the vocalization of speech to an area in the frontal lobe, and the comprehension of speech to the parietal. In the sensory and motor cortex there is a high degree of topography with different zones dedicated to sensation and movement in different parts of the body, with poor representation for the leg and foot, more for the arm and hand, and most for the face. This topographic anatomy, the dedication of certain areas to specific functions, is lacking only in two cortical areas, the extreme frontal, known as the prefrontal cortex, and the cingulate gyrus, cortical tissue tucked deep within the hemispheric cleft. These cortical areas have no clear-cut topographic anatomy nor do they demonstrate any specific executive function. They are the apex of our second brain.

The subcortical brain lacks the distinctive convoluted architecture of the cortex. It consists of aggregates of cell bodies deep beneath the surface. These extend from the brain stem, the point where the spinal cord enters the cranium, and expand in size and scope as they reach the cingulate and prefrontal cortex. It is, in cellular volume, less than the size of a woman's fist. The predominant neurotransmitters, quite unlike those of the cortex, are serotonin, noradrenaline, and dopamine. The subcortical brain is the vegetative, emotional, memorizing, thoughtful, and behavioral brain. It is soft-wired. Subcortical neurons are more complicated than those in the cortex. They are capable of many reactions. Their response to provocation is much less predictable than those in the cortex. Subcortical neurons have choice.

Vegetative functions, those we share with all mammals, are organized at the base of the subcortical brain. Visceral and cardiac activity are controlled by the autonomic system. Controlled by other systems are wakefulness, sleep, appetite, and the perception of pain. The ability to temper and modulate pain is a fundamental attribute of our existence, and it is no evolutionary accident that analgesic centers lie at the brain base where they intermingle with nerve tracts carrying painful signals up from the spinal cord. Nor is it an accident that they are proximate in location to that brain area known as the *locus ceruleus*. These cells, with predominant gamma-amniobutyric acid transmitters, are the brain's center for the control of vigilance and attention (uncontrolled vigilance is the clinical disorder we know as anxiety). In the upper brain stem is the hypothalamus. Located above the pituitary gland, it employs for its actions dopamine and other neurotransmitters known as hormones. These subserve the control of metabolic energy by the release of thyroid and adrenal hormones and of sexual energy by the release of gonadal hormones. In the hypothalamus also are control systems for the body's rhythms. These range from our diurnal rhythms to our lunar, seasonal, and annual rhythms. Above the hypothalamus are the thalamus, the site where pain becomes a conscious experience, and the basal ganglia where movement is controlled. Forward of this is a spread-eagle array of nerve cells known as the limbic system. It is the repository of experiential memories and is the agency of thought. At the apex of the limbic system are the cingulate and prefrontal cortex. These are the great incorporators. There all our vegetative, emotional, and behavioral functions are organized into that supreme expression of our being, our personality. Accordingly, it is these two areas that have been and still are the object of psychosurgery, formerly prefrontal lobotomy for extreme disorders of behavior, and more currently cingulotomy for the treatment of refractory disorders of personality such as obsessive-compulsive disorder and, rarely, for that derangement of behavior we call chronic pain (it occasionally works!). The subcortical brain is the control brain, the assimilative, organizational, emotional, social, and sometimes painful brain. Endowed with choice, and lacking specific executive function, it is less lateralized, less topographic than the cortex. It has more important things to do.

Each of our control brain functions, from the most primitive to the most complex, may disorder into clinical expression.

Autonomic control may disorder into altered gastrointestinal
motility, the irritable bowel syndrome, or into that painful disorder
of regional blood flow we know as reflex sympathetic dystrophy.
Analgesic control may disorder into migraine or chronic painfulness and vigilance control into anxiety. Feeding and appetite may
disorder into obesity or anorexia-bulimia, and sleep-wake into
insomnia or narcolepsy. Mood control may disorder into depression or mania and thought into delusions, obsessions, or
schizophrenic psychosis. And in that most remarkable of subcortical diseases, the control and integration of personality is
disordered into multiple personality disorder.

All these clinical expressions have a number of attributes in
common. Many are genetically based and have a familial incidence.
Migraine, depression, bipolar disease, and substance abuse are often
inherited as are occasionally schizophrenia and personality disorders. Some, including migraine, depression, and chronic pain occur
after cerebral injury, be this head trauma, stroke, or meningitis.
Many bear a strong relationship to emotional stress. Depression
and schizophrenia certainly do. Migraine and other states of
painfulness also. Hyperthyroidism, an uncontrolled release of
hypothalamic hormones, occasionally appears after emotional
stress. The examples are endless.

Many subcortical diseases are periodic. The most common,
of course, is luteal phase mood disorder, a lunar period disease
commonly known as the premenstrual syndrome. Another disorder
of discernible periodicity is seasonal affective disorder. This is an
annual depression seemingly dictated by the short light days of
winter. A diurnal pattern of periodicity is operative in that form of
migraine known as cluster headaches. Attacks of severe eye and face
pain occur principally, and in some cases exclusively, at night. Cluster
headache is a remarkable example of periodicity. A siege of recurring
headaches may last for weeks and then disappear to recur, sometimes
seasonally, but more often randomly, sometimes years later.

Depression, mania, and migraine, as well as some other states of
painfulness, are recurrent diseases. Sometimes they obey compre-
hensible diurnal, lunar, seasonal, or annual rhythms, but they often

appear in a temporal array quite beyond our understanding. They are the expression of a biologic disorder, an alternate configuration of the serotonin-noradrenaline-dopamine axis in the subcortical brain. Most are slow diseases. They don't appear overnight. They are attended by a gradual evolution, appearing in fragments before the full disease is manifest. (Migraine, which is hardwired and genetically dictated, is an exception.) They represent a gradual shift of the neural apparatus into an alternate channel, and it is no coincidence that the drugs we employ for these disorders, the antipsychotics, the SSRIs, and the tricyclics are themselves slow drugs. They do not exert an immediate pharmacologic effect. Their onset of action is measured in many days. This is the requisite time required for them to work.

The cerebral cortex is hard-wired, quick-acting, and highly integrated in the interdependent functioning of vision, audition, tactile sensation, and movement. Our subcortical brain is softer-wired and slower-acting, but its actions are similarly interdependent and integrated. The assembly of sleep, appetite, mood, energy, temperament, behavior, and the perception of pain cannot be viewed as isolated and separate functions. They are too interactive for that. Thus, an encounter with a stressful life event (be this a job change, the death of a loved one, or a painful fracture of bone) will provoke and challenge the entirety of the subcortical system. Its disarray may manifest as change in appetite, depressed mood, anxiety, or a change in biologic rhythms with disordered sleep or disordered menstruation. These effects are usually transient. The resiliency and redundancy of our neural systems, that is the integrity of our infrastructure, allow us most of the time to compensate for destructive life experiences. Sometimes, however, our capacity for control is overwhelmed and the subcortical system reroutes in its entirety or at least some large fragment of its entirety into the clinical expression of psychiatric illness. This evolution occurs over an interval of many days or weeks with the gradual appearance of fragments, partials, and *formes fruste*. Only late in the game do they become full-blown, recognizable psychiatric diseases, and even then there is usually a mixture. We recognize these as comorbidities. Anxiety disorder, for example, is often comorbid with depression. Substance abuse is comorbid with both anxiety and depression. Painfulness, certainly, is comorbid with depression and substance abuse. Much as we would like it, pure, unalloyed, distinctive neuropsychiatric entities almost never exist.

Depression is the paradigm of neuropsychiatric illness. It is a disorder of mood characterized by hopelessness, despondency, and symbolically by self-hate, but there is more to it than that. Depression is associated, as are all psychiatric disorders, with a reconfiguration in the entirety of the subcortical system. Thus, depression is attended by clinical expressions, both behavioral and biologic, almost infinite in their variety. Autonomic function is disordered. Both constipation and the irritable bowel syndrome are common in the depressive. The control of appetite sufficient for the maintenance of energy is disassembled into weight loss or obesity. Sleep, a function of diurnal rhythms, is almost invariably disarrayed. Attention and anxiolysis are disturbed with the appearance of apathy and sometimes of hyperactivity, restlessness, and anxiety. The integrity of analgesic systems is disordered, thus the common occurrence of painfulness and migraine in the depressive. Cognition and memory are disturbed, a phenomenon known as the pseudode-mentia of depression. The integrity of thought is disassembled, and obsessions, delusions, and in some cases psychosis ensue. Even the organization of motor activity is disarrayed with the develop-ment of postural change and in extreme cases catatonia, a fixed, immobile posture. Sexual drive is disrupted with diminished libido, impotence, and anorgasmia. Impulse control is lost with behavioral disinhibition and suicidal ideation. The control of memory is disassembled and remote experiences are recruited uncomfortably to consciousness.

Depression is not just a disorder of mood. It represents, in its full expression, a total disassembly of the vegetative and behavioral brain. Depressed mood is simply the predominant display. But sometimes not. Odell's depression manifested as violent, aggressive behavior. Michelle's as the pain of a brachial plexus injury. The hair-dresser discussed in chapter four manifested her depression as tension headaches and Harriet, believe it or not, as pain, insomnia, weight loss, and pericarditis.

Fragments, partials, *formes frustes*, and comorbidities. Psychiatric illnesses, virtually all of them, overlap and coexist to an extent that most of the time it is impossible to achieve a precise, encompassing diagnosis. This is the reason psychiatrists, all of them, recognize that in the treatment of their patients, achieving an absolutely correct diagnosis is much less important than finding a drug that works. This is certainly the case with chronic pain.

Painfulness, as a disease entity, can only be understood, as depression can only be understood, as a derangement of multiple subcortical functions of which disordered analgesia is but one expression. Appetite is disrupted with weight gain or loss. Motor systems are disordered with the development of abnormal movements, restless legs. Sexual activity is diminished with lack of sexual desire and impotence. Attention is disordered with apathy or restlessness and hyperactivity. Mood is disassembled into depression and thought into obsessions. Gratification systems lose their normal inhibition, and drug dependency and addiction develop. Behavior becomes intemperate and irascible, and ultimately that most inviolate of our attributes, personality, is fractured. "I am just not the same person I was before I became painful."

Depression is not just a disorder of mood. It represents, in its full expression, a total disassembly of the vegetative and behavioral brain.

Sleep is disordered—always sleep. There is something very strange about the way our subcortical brains work, something that is counter-intuitive. We share with all mammals as a fundamental biologic attribute the integration of sleep, wakefulness, and appetite. Foraging and rest and their successful assembly are necessary for the simple maintenance of metabolic energy. It all begins there. Everything else is an add-on. The most complex add-on up the evolutionary and developmental scale is the creation of personality. Our personalities are unique, so far as we know, in the universe. Our vegetative functions, on the other hand, we share with

most other mammals. We should reasonably expect vegetative functions to be constant and virtually immutable, and our personalities
on the other end of the scale to be fragile and easily disarrayed. It
doesn't work that way. Our personalities are highly resistant to fluctuation and change, whereas our primordial functions of sleep and
appetite are fragile and easily subject to disassembly. So contrary to
common sense, disordered sleep and appetite are among the most
sensitive barometers of neurobiologic disintegration.

Many years ago we recognized that painful patients were often
depressed. With the advent of the tricyclic drugs we observed that
painfulness responded to antidepressant therapy. Thus, in our
search for a simple answer to a complex problem, we ascribed a
state of pain to a state of depression. That is all gone by the board
now. Tricyclic drugs do work for pain, but SSRIs don't, and many
painful patients, we have learned, are not depressed. Now we have
gone to the other side of the scale, and in our search for some
coherence, some understanding of painfulness, we have come to
view it as an entity separate from depression. Nearly every medical
text states that the analgesic effect of the tricyclics is independent
of their antidepressant effect—*and the texts are clearly wrong*.
Painfulness cannot be viewed as a distinct and isolated entity. It is
no more a thing unto itself than is depression, substance abuse,
post-traumatic stress disorder, bipolar disease, or any other
neuropsychiatric illness. They, along with painfulness, form a
continuum, and each of them in their display overlap and coexist
with the others. They are comorbid, just as fibromyalgia, chronic
headache, the failed back, and reflex sympathetic dystrophy are
comorbid, overlapping with each other in their clinical exhibition.

CHAPTER NINE

Sexual Abuse

A cute pain is the product of corporal injury. Chronic pain is the product of the mind. It comes, most of the time, to those whose cerebral function has been altered by destructive life experiences. Sometimes the stressor appears proximate in time to the development of pain. The loss of a job, the loss of a loved one, a major infectious illness, or a stroke can all generate painfulness as their aftermath. Equally often, the stressor is remote in time. Past depression or past pharmacologic experiences may evolve months or years later into chronic pain. There is another remote experience which, more predictably than any other, incites a life of chronic pain, and that is childhood abuse, particularly sexual abuse. The subject is disturbing, and many readers, certainly those who have suffered the experience, will find it distressing. This is regrettable but unavoidable. It is quite impossible to understand the nature and meaning of chronic pain without addressing the issue.

Sexual abuse may occur as a single brutal event, a rape. Perhaps even more destructively, it occurs under persuasion and is repetitive, sometimes ritualistic. Surprisingly, it may mimic tenderness, this in the form of fondling. Regardless, the stain is often ineradicable, and the victim is left with guilt, remorse, and frightening flashbacks that may last a lifetime. The frequency of sexual abuse in the chronically painful female (less the male) is astonishing. This is particularly so in those whose pain begins in their youth or early maturity.

Patsy was chubby, typical for a painful patient. She was also coy and charming—perhaps less typical. After a few preliminaries in which she described the chronic pain in her neck, shoulders, and upper back, and the sensitive trigger points, I inquired about her sleep. Her legs were restless, and she had difficulty finding a position of comfort at night. She suffered frequent painful awakenings, and her sleep was never restorative. She had been obese most of her thirty years. She occasionally dieted successfully, but was never able to sustain weight loss. She suffered chronic headaches as well as fibromyalgia and used opiates regularly. She acknowledged her moodiness with intervals of depression beginning as a teenager. When I asked if there was a history of abuse, her speech and mannerisms changed. Her voice assumed a higher pitch, and she regressed into a child. She gestured with her hands and talked about her home on the farm and her dog, Fuzzy. He slept beside her bed every night and walked with her to the school bus stop each morning. He was there in the afternoon when she returned. He was a spaniel and a very smart dog, she emphasized. He was her best friend. Then she smiled, a visage I did not like at all, and returned to her prior personality. Her voice and manners assumed their original structure, and she said, "I frighten you, don't I?"

Multiple personality disorder is usually the product of childhood trauma, most commonly sexual abuse. In Patsy's case, it was repetitive and candle-lit ritualistic. It began about age five as best she could remember, and lasted until she got married at age sixteen to get away.

There are few diseases as destructive as that imposed by childhood abuse. Its manifold effects have been listed before, but they're worth repeating. Victims suffer irregular sleep throughout their lives. They are appetite-irregular. Most are obese, but some experience the anorexia-bulimia syndrome. Their mood is labile with rapid swings and recurrent depression. They suffer anxiety and are subject to exaggerated behaviors in response to emotional or physical stimuli. Conversion reaction is by no means rare. Painfulness is a very common expression of the disorder. Headache, fibromyalgia, irritable bowel syndrome, and the premenstrual syndrome occur with great frequency. The most profound product of childhood sexual abuse is multiple personality disorder. In the big scheme of things, however, it is a rather rare disease. It is but a single, albeit the most dramatic, manifestation of the syndrome of childhood abuse. It is the tip of the iceberg. Much more common is the maldevelopment of other subcortical systems. The sexually abused are denied any semblance of regularity and control in their behavior and their biology. This may be the reason why, unable to control their own lives, they sometimes attempt to control others. This is exactly what happened when Patsy said after her disassociation into a child, "I frighten you, don't I?" It was an attempt to establish dominance, control, over her physician. An unpleasant and highly maladaptive behavior, it is one reason, among many, why victims of abuse can be so difficult to treat. Their relationships with others, whether friends or physicians, are sometimes confrontational and manipulative.

Many abused patients come, not surprisingly, from dysfunctional homes. They frequently have a family history of depression and quite often of bipolar disease. They also have a family history of alcoholism. Thus, these unfortunate people suffer a double hit. Both genetics and malnurture are operative in their illness. No wonder at all that they tend to have uncomfortable lives and relationships. They are distrustful, perhaps understandably, and they are often uncooperative patients. They flit from one doctor to another presenting bizarre symptoms and extravagant behaviors. This is the reason they so frequently acquire exotic diagnoses. If you go to enough doctors with enough strange complaints, sooner or later you will acquire an exotic diagnosis. Porphyria, multiple sclerosis, and lupus erythematosus are examples. These are all fashionable and politically correct diseases. Each is associated with a high incidence of painfulness and, as every physician recognizes, a variety of unusual emotional behaviors.

Porphyria, multiple sclerosis, and lupus all have uncertain clinical boundaries and in some cases represent very subjective diagnoses, not always easily confirmable by laboratory examination. These diagnoses, perhaps sometimes derived inappropriately, legitimize the patients' painfulness and behavior on the basis of their disease.

No harm at all in that. Their pain and their behavior are legitimate symptoms of disease, but quite frequently they are not due to porphyria, multiple sclerosis, or lupus. They are the product of sexual abuse, and I wish that physicians would simply include in their interrogations the question of childhood abuse. They would be astonished by the frequency of this experience in their difficult and treatment-resistant patients.

It is remarkable how well many victims of abuse manage to get by. I respect and admire them enormously. Some achieve stable marriages and manage to hold responsible jobs and to raise children, but they are rarely happy or contented people. Painful childhood experiences never go away.

Karen consulted many physicians regarding her chronic pain. Most of them told her she had fibromyalgia. A few suggested that the problem was mental and that she needed psychotherapy. Only one, among a dozen or so, offered a diagnosis she accepted as credible—lupus erythematosus. An unpleasant disease to be sure, but certainly a more honorable one than imaginary pain. Karen embraced therapy with the drugs Methotrexate and Plaquenil. They can be very helpful in the treatment of inflammatory arthritis, be this due to rheumatoid disease or lupus. Their clinical effect, however, is slow, and benefit is measured not in days or weeks, but in months. Two years into her treatment, Karen remained as painful as before. The drugs had not helped.

She was willing to talk about her past history, medical and personal (painful patients often are—they need to talk). At age ten, Karen fell under the persuasion of a teenage cousin who demanded, under threat, the performance of oral sex. The acts ended after a few months but irreparable damage had been done. Karen was forever scarred, emotionally and biologically. Did she really have lupus? You figure.

Many victims accommodate to their experience by employing denial. The horror and shame are relegated to subconsciousness. Sooner or later, though, it all comes back.

Sarah was lifelong obese and painful. She remembered only fragments of her childhood, but this was never a bother until she entered a diet clinic and heard a lecture on obesity as a product of childhood sexual abuse. Hearing that, she remembered the old man who lived next door. He always seemed to be there when she went to pick up the mail. One day he invited her into his home for chocolate. He stripped and fondled and masturbated on her. When she told me this, she stood up and faced away. She told her story to the wall.

Peggy was a smoker. Seeking a cure for her addiction, she consulted a therapist who employed hypnosis. Under hypnotic suggestion she was carried back to the time when she began using cigarettes. She awoke from her trance tearful and agitated. Her habit—and her stepfather's molestations—had begun at the same time. That experience had been forgotten, repressed into subconsciousness, until released by hypnosis. Her discovery did not help her stop smoking. It only made her fibromyalgia worse.

I wish that physicians would simply include in their interrogations the question of childhood abuse. They would be astonished by the frequency of this experience in their difficult and treatment-resistant patients.

Melinda grew up in a prosperous home. She was forced repetitively into sexual acts by her two older brothers. It began at age seven and extended into her early teens. As is typically, and unfortunately, the case, she never told. The shame was too great. Melinda entered maturity— and denial. She married well and had children. She told me later, in one of her few moments of candor, that she had always known that things weren't quite right. She suffered unaccountable depressive intervals and periodic attacks of anxiety. She could never figure it out, she said, until the occasion of her daughter's seventh birthday party. At that celebration, commemorating the same age at which her assaults had begun, it all came back. Beyond repression, the experience returned to consciousness, and she entered a sustained depression. Within a short while she developed excruciating pain in her back and legs. A ruptured lumbar disc was suspect, but her imaging studies were all normal. None of the several neurosurgeons and neurologists who examined her could explain her pain. Melinda is now a spinal cripple, wheelchair-bound, paralyzed and unable to move her lower extremities—a conversion reaction. She remains depressed, sleepless, painful, opiate-dependent, and in denial. She is immune to any suggestion that her illness represents a product of her remote experiences. "I have pinched nerves in my back," she says, "don't you see how paralyzed I am."

Agnes was referred for treatment of her failed back. She suffered a lumbar disc herniation with sciatica. Her operation was reasonably straight-forward. The disc was removed and pressure on the nerve relieved, but she did not recover. As is nearly always the case in the chroni-cally painful, her symptoms could not be disassembled from her life experiences and memories. Her sciatica, a random act of nature, occurred at an unfortunate time in her life (few diseases occur at fortunate times). Her symptoms began about the time she discovered that her mother, her dearest friend, had inoperable cancer and was dying. Agnes deferred her surgery in order to care for her mother. She hung on for several months as a painful caregiver, but her sciatica progressively worsened. Her neurosurgeon implored her to have an operation. The likelihood of success was great, he thought, and after a fairly short convalescence she could return and provide more fitting care for her mother. The disc was removed, but the pain was not. When her mother died a few weeks later, Agnes experienced enor-mous grief. She entered a sustained and destructive depression. Her erratic sleep became even more disturbed, and she began to experi-ence, at midlife, bed-wetting.

Enuresis is common in children—usually in boys, less in girls. What it means we really don't know. It doesn't seem to carry any major aftermath. It almost always goes away in the early teens. Agnes was enuretic in her childhood. It had been a pattern of behavior for many years, but it disappeared, at least until she entered her depression. It recurred then, very plausibly the recrudescence of a remote behavioral memory.

As I interviewed Agnes, her attachment to her mother and her grief over her loss were clearly evident. I asked about her father. She never felt like she knew him very well, and his death, several years before, never affected her very much. I continued my questions, and she responded with the litany of lifelong disordered sleep and moodiness. She didn't particularly enjoy the company of men, and she had never married. I asked her what her childhood was like, and she replied that she didn't remember much of it except that she was unhappy as a youngster.

"Were you ever physically or sexually abused?"

"I don't know. I think probably I was."

"What do you mean, 'probably'?"

"I remember that when I wet the bed at night, someone would come in to change the sheets." She paused.

"And?"

"Sometimes when I woke up in the morning, I would hurt."

"In your genitals?"

"Yes, and one time—I am pretty sure about this—I remember something big and warm over me and close, pressing me very hard."

"Who was it?"

"I don't know."

Joan sprained her back lifting a typewriter. She was treated with Ultram, but failed to recover. Her pain progressed to involve her neck and shoulders. It was incessant, and it kept her from sleeping at night. Her physician suspected that she had fibromyalgia. He prescribed Amitriptyline and referred her to me.

"Tell me about yourself, Joan."

"I am thirty-five years old, and I am a piano teacher. I have been married for ten years to a fine man, and I have two children."

"Did you have any problem with pain before you developed fibromyalgia?"

"Yes, I've had tension headaches and endometriosis, but they were nothing compared to this fibromyalgia."

"You have been taking Amitriptyline for a couple of weeks now. Has it helped?"

"Yes, the pain is a little bit better, but I still don't sleep very well at all."

"How long have you had trouble sleeping?"

"I have never slept well, but it really got bad when I developed fibromyalgia. The pain keeps me awake at night."

"Sometimes people with insomnia have a lot of muscle jerkings at night. Do you have anything like that?"

"I certainly do. Whenever I try to go to sleep, my legs start moving about. I can't hold them still."

"That's called restless legs. It is a good name, isn't it?"

"Yes, a very good name. My legs have been restless for a long time. Sometimes even during the day, I can't hold them still."

"Are you depressed?"

"Yes, I'll admit, I am. The pain would make anybody depressed."

"Have you ever suffered depression in the past?"

"Yes, whenever my headaches or endometriosis flared up, I would get very depressed."

"Did you ever take medicine for it?"

"Not until I got started on Amitriptyline. I understand that is a medicine for depression."

"That's correct, but it is also useful for chronic pain, whether you are depressed or not."

"That's good to know. I wondered about that."

"Do you mind telling me what your childhood was like? Were you happy as a kid?"

"Yes, I was very happy. Why in the world do you ask that question?"

"I hope I haven't offended you, but I usually ask. Many people with chronic pain have a history of childhood trauma. Some of them have suffered sexual abuse."

She hesitated and then said, "Well, there is something I suppose I need to tell you then. I was raped when I was in college."

"Do you mind telling me about it?"

"I was walking to the library one Friday night, and a man grabbed me and threw me into his car. He drove me to a cabin in the woods and locked me in a room. He had his way with me through the weekend, and then he drove me back to the campus and let me out."

"Did you report it to the authorities?"

"No, I had some acquaintances who had been raped, and reporting it never did them any good."

"You never sought counseling?"

"No, my friends helped me through it. I gradually got over it."

"Do you ever flashback to it?"

"Yes, I used to have nightmares, and even now a certain sight or sound or smell will bring it back to me."

"How often do you have the flashbacks?"

"At first I had a lot of them, but over the years they have mostly gone away. Recently, though, they are coming back."

"When did that actually happen?"

"A few months ago."

"When your fibromyalgia began?"

"Yes, that's when they came back. I think I see where you are trying to go with this. Do you really think my rape has anything to do with my fibromyalgia? How could this possibly be? It was over fifteen years ago!"

"I can't answer that question. I will just offer you my opinion, and you can draw your own conclusions. I suspect that the trauma you experienced was so overwhelming that it actually altered the way your brain works. Look at it this way—since that event your brain has been hypervigilant to some sights, sounds, and smells. I believe your brain is also hypervigilant to another sensation, that of pain. That is why you developed fibromyalgia from your muscle sprain, and I suspect it may have something to do with your painful headaches and endometriosis."

"Are you saying that my pain is coming from my mind, that I am imagining it?"

"Yes, I believe that pain is coming from your mind, but it is certainly not an imagination. Let me ask you this. Are your flash-backs some kind of imagination?"

"No! The flashbacks are real, and they are horrible. It is like I am being raped again. There is nothing imaginary about them."

"Nor is there anything imaginary about your pain. It is the product of chemistry within your mind. And we have drugs that can alter that chemistry. Amitriptyline is one of them, and it is already beginning to help you. I am going to increase the dose and add another drug called Klonopin. I am pretty sure you will continue to get better and, as you do, I think you will find that your pain and flashbacks will pretty much go away together."

"Oh my God! You mean if I had taken medicines many years ago, I wouldn't be having the flashbacks?"

"Probably not, and I doubt that you would have been so sleepless and depressed. Nor, I suspect, would you have been so painful. It's even possible that you might not have restless legs."

"You are giving me a lot to think about."

"I know. I am not asking that you buy into it quite yet, but I do ask that you take the medicines I prescribe."

"I will certainly do that."

"Another question, if I may?"

"Yes, go ahead."

"Have you ever told any of your doctors about the rape?"

"No, you are the only doctor who ever invited me to talk about it."

CHAPTER TEN

Referred Pain

Helen's pain began at age seventeen. Her menstrual cramps, until then a minor bother, became severe. Laparoscopic surgery identified endometriosis. Intrauterine tissue had migrated about the pelvis and, under hormonal control, swelled and became painful during menstruation. The aberrant tissue was removed, but there was benefit for only a short while. Pain, which had initially occurred only during menstruation, became incessant. Hormonal therapy was ineffective. Another laparoscopic operation to remove abnormal tissue was performed but with even less success than with the first. Helen was incapacitated with pain, and at age twenty-five, unmarried and childless, she consented to a hysterectomy and pelvic clean-out. She was advised that this operation, the definitive therapy, would relieve her pain.

Immediately on awakening from anesthesia, at the first instant of consciousness, Helen experienced severe pain in her back and lower extremities. The consultants were reined in and, as is typical with the painful patient, the diagnostic and therapeutic interventions began once more. Her lumbar MRI suggested multiple disc bulges. She was treated with an epidural steroid infusion, the injection of cortisone into soft tissues of the back, bathing the inflamed nerves as they exit the vertebral column. It helped a bit at first. Cortisone, after all, will help almost anything for a while. The injections were repeated over the course of several weeks, but they became less and less effective. Myelography, the injection of radiographic contrast material into the spinal canal, confirmed the disc bulges. They were plausibly, but by no means certainly, the cause of her pain. (Many people have bulging discs and no pain at all, just as many have endometriosis and no pain.) She came to a lumbar laminectomy and removal of the offending discs, but her pain did not go away. The failed pelvis had become the failed back. Next (there is often a next), a spinal fusion to stabilize a back now somewhat bent by her discectomy. A heroic and definitive procedure, it didn't work.

Helen's remarkable history represented no chain of coincidence, of that I was sure. The astonishing pattern of recurrent pain, of repetitive failure to recover, simply could not be ascribed to chance. Would that some physician somewhere along the way had gone to the trouble to obtain a proper history.

Helen was gang-raped at age sixteen. Her painful dysmenorrhea began shortly thereafter. Endometriosis, a common cause of dysmenorrhea, was identified. Surgical removal of the abnormal tissue did not, however, relieve her pain. It is not difficult to remove aberrant endometrial tissue, but it is quite difficult to remove a painful memory. With each menstruation, the memory was kindled. It acquired a life of its own. A neural routing predicated on prior experiences changed from an occasional to a dominant behavior, and Helen entered a life of painfulness. We can be sure she had an organic disease, endometriosis, but was it really the cause of her pain? No, it was the agency of her pain, not the cause of it. Hysterectomy didn't cure Helen's pain. It simply moved it to an adjacent part of the body. One does not rupture a lumbar disc as one lies immobilized on the operating table. The unlikelihood of this coincidence is staggering. Sure, she had bulging discs, but were they the cause of her back pain?

Helen responded rather well to tricyclic drug therapy, and I think there is a reasonable understanding why she did. Her rape occurred when she was sixteen, certainly a precious, formative age in her life, but not so precious and formative as age seven. She had sufficient time before the trauma for her subcortical brain to assemble its function in good order. She had an infrastructure of wellness. That is why she got well.

In most mind-soul diseases, it is quite impossible to identify an absolute reduction in this or that neurotransmitter. Their treatment does not involve replacing something that is missing. Rather, it involves the rearrangement of complex systems involving millions of cells back into adaptive from maladaptive behaviors. Helen responded to drug therapy. To ascribe her improvement, however, simply to the alteration of neurochemistry is, I believe, to miss the boat. What happened, miraculously, was that the drugs rendered inoperative and unneeded a maladaptive routing and resurrected an adaptive one. Her painfulness improved substantially and her depression also. Helen will probably never be a truly vivacious and happy person (painful childhood experiences never go away), but she may, with drug therapy, experience a life of relative comfort and productivity.

They don't all do so well, and for good reason. The sexually abused person whose experience dates from the very youthful preteen years fails to acquire an integrated system of biology and behavior. There is no infrastructure of wellness. Nothing to fall back on. This is the reason pharmacotherapy for pain, remarkably effective in most patients, is less so in painful states generated by early childhood sexual abuse. Drugs don't incite new patterns of neurotransmitter activity. They merely restore the old ones.

Nerve fibers from the sacral and pelvic area enter the spinal cord at its lowest level and ascend in tracts into the brain. Fibers from the low back and lower extremities enter next, and they are layered over those from the pelvis. Then, in sequence, fibers from the abdomen, thorax, upper extremities, and the head and face are progressively added in laminar form. This layering, altered only slightly along the way, extends into the brain. Axons carrying tactile sensation are destined to end in the parietal cortex, and those carrying pain in the thalamus. The cortex is highly topographic and, therefore, the perception of tactile sensation is acute. We can easily discriminate two separate points of touch on our fingertips. We could not begin to discriminate two separate points of pain on our fingers. The thalamus, that portion of the sub-cortical brain which processes pain, is less topographic than the cortex. It lacks the ability to discriminate. Therefore, the perception of pain is subject to anatomic confusion. Pain is poorly localized. It is diffuse and it spreads, and unlike any other sensory experience, it may be referred away from its site of origin.

Pain begins as an electrochemical message in the peripheral nerves. It is propagated upwards until it reaches the thalamus and there becomes a conscious experience. Along that short but neurophysiologically slow journey (painful signals travel more slowly than tactile ones), the electrochemical message is modulated by analgesic centers. These have processed other pains and recorded them, we can be sure, in the form of memory. Could these memories be recruited into the conscious perception of pain and its referral to other body parts? It certainly happened in the man with coronary artery disease. He felt his cardiac pain only at the site of his remote back fracture. Could the memory of a peptic ulcer influence the perception of cardiac pain into the abdomen? Or a rotator cuff injury into the shoulder, or an abscessed tooth into the jaw? Helen experienced severe back pain on referral from her pelvis. Was that not, in the endgame, the product of an experiential memory?

CHAPTER ELEVEN

Reflex Sympathetic Dystrophy

R eflex sympathetic dystrophy (RSD) is the most dreadful of the painful diseases. In no other illness is the physician so called upon to *do something*—even if it is wrong.

A painful injury, usually in an extremity, incites an unusual reaction. It recruits the autonomic nervous system, that subcortical apparatus dedicated to the control of blood flow, into misbehavior. Blood vessels constrict. Muscles wither and contract. Bones becomes osteoporotic, and the skin glossy, atrophic, and cold. As with other states of chronic pain, sleep, appetite, and mood are all disordered, but the predominant and most visible effect is reduction in blood flow and with it extravagant pain. Why a painful injury should occasionally incite the autonomic system into dysfunction is problematic. It may have something to do with age and gender because reflex sympathetic dystrophy is usually a disease of young women.

Luz, just graduated from high school, found employment in a grocery store. There only a short while, she slipped on a wet place and broke her left ankle. The fracture was set in the emergency room. In a few days her foot began to swell. The orthopedist replaced the cast and noted that her pulse was bounding, but that her foot was cool and blanched.

Luz's fracture, even though immobilized by her cast, became progressively painful and kept her awake at night. She began to experience hyperpathic pain. Merely touching the tips of her toes was uncomfortable to her. X-rays showed satisfactory healing of the fracture, but when the cast was removed, the ankle and foot were cadaveric in appearance. Luz's pain was severe and incessant.

Nerve cells are resilient. They have the inherent capacity to reconfigure and change their function, a phenomenon known as *neural plasticity*. Old cells learn new tricks. Fortunately so, for this is the reason we recover from strokes and other neural injuries. Nature's flexibility, however, is not always adaptive. Sometimes it leads to the brain attacking the body, and this is what occurs in reflex sympathetic dystrophy. The capacity of the brain to actually wither an extremity challenges credulity. But it happens, and by a mechanism we have not yet begun to understand.

That segment of the autonomic nervous system known as the *sympathetic* is housed in the brain stem, and axons from its cells descend and exit the spinal cord throughout its length to synapse (communicate) with other neurons in aggregates known as sympathetic ganglia. These lie adjacent to the vertebral column. Nerve fibers from these ganglia course in company with blood vessels throughout the body and control their reactivity. This, so far as we know, is their sole function. By virtue of their plasticity, however, they can, under provocation, reconfigure and actually generate pain.

Luz was treated with a sympathetic block. A needle was introduced into her back and directed to the ganglia along the lumbar spine. An anesthetic was injected, denying sympathetic innervation and the power of vasoconstriction to her extremity. As predictably happens, her leg, formerly cold and moist, became warm and dry. Her pain diminished, but it reappeared, as did coldness, when the anesthetic wore off. The blocks were repeated several days running in an attempt to somehow arrest her disease. With each injection her leg would warm and her pain partially abate.

Encouraged by the response, her physicians elected to do a sympathectomy. The ganglia were surgically removed, and Luz's lower extremity was deprived of sympathetic innervation. The vessels dilated and blood flow was restored. We used to treat high blood pressure with sympathectomy. It was an awkward form of treatment, but it worked pretty well because it forever denied the blood vessels the capacity to constrict. Not so with Luz. A plastic nervous system endowed with the capacity to change its function cannot be easily contained, even by surgical ablation. A few days after her operation, her leg again became cold and very painful. God alone knows how this can happen.

Luz's toes contracted into deformity, their nails piercing and inflaming the skin. It was impossible to clean these wounds. The application of soap and water was painful, and anesthesia was required to even clip the nails. Luz's leg had become inanimate, dirty, dank, and smelly. She required high level opiate therapy, Demerol (probably not the best drug, but commonly used), every three or four hours, day and night.

Luz accepted amputation. She was told by her physicians that the operation might not relieve her pain, but it was warranted, however, simply as a matter of hygiene. Whatever pain relief she achieved would be a welcome bonus. The limb was amputated below the knee, and Luz was rendered, if not painless, at least clean. She developed phantom limb pain. She continued to feel her nails piercing her flesh, an experiential memory.

Pain can sometimes be relieved or abated by a counter stimulus. If we bump our knee, we rub it forcefully or even scratch it, and that sensation will, at least for a while, override the pain. Thus, a treatment form known as transcutaneous electrical nerve stimulation (TENS). An electrode over a painful area, connected to a battery, provides an electrical stimulation to the skin, and a mild shock or buzz replaces the pain with a less distressful sensation. In cases of severe pain, the stimulator can be placed not on the skin but on the surface of the spinal cord itself. An electrode is placed above the dorsal columns of the spinal cord, that segment of spinal architecture dedicated to the mediation of sensation from the body to the brain. The dorsal columns are laminated, and those nerve fibers most recently arrived in the spinal cord lie closest to the surface. Thus, in theory, an electrical stimulus applied to the spinal cord at the appropriate level overrides the painful signal. A dorsal column stimulator works some of the time, but it didn't work in Luz. Her pain continued.

It was time for another operation, the cauterization of spinal areas adjacent to the sensory nerve roots, the dorsal root entry zone (DREZ) procedure. Luz's spinal cord was surgically exposed and a portion of it selectively destroyed, hopefully to remove forever the capacity of her brain to receive a painful signal from the upper extremity. It failed miserably. Her pain was not relieved, and the cauterization and manipulation of the dorsal roots and their adjacent ganglia invoked a biologic memory. The zoster virus, the infective agent in Luz's remote chicken pox, was sequestered in those ganglia. The virus was activated by the DREZ procedure and Luz developed shingles. The rash and pain extended over her buttock and leg down to her stump. With time, the rash went away but she failed to recover. Luz developed postherpetic neuralgia and her pain, formerly confined to her missing leg, extended into her hip and back. She had become quarter body painful. She had reflex sympathetic dystrophy, phantom limb pain, and postherpetic neuralgia. There were all comorbid.

When her disease began, Luz lost all desire for food or sleep. She had no sense of appetite. She would only pick at her meals. She had no need for sleep. During her hospitalizations she was observed to take only occasional catnaps. All through the night she would sit with the nurses, wakeful and reactive, chatting and sharing cigarettes. Luz's diurnal rhythms were totally ablated. There was no day-night, sleep-wake harmony, but her other rhythms, notably the lunar, were unaffected. The pattern of her menstruation changed not at all through her ordeal. Such is the capacity of the subcortical brain to express its disorders incompletely, in fragments and partials. Our subcortical brain, remember, has choice.

Nature had another trick to play on Luz. Some three years or so into her illness, she began to experience spontaneous pain in her right side, first in the hip, then the leg, and finally the foot. Not so severe at first, it gradually became more of a problem. Her good leg became cold, sweaty, and ultimately hyperpathic. Her RSD had attacked the opposite member. A powerful, dominant neural assembly in Luz's subcortical brain could not by the force of its energy remain spatially isolated, just as it could not remain behaviorally isolated. The pressure was simply too great. The spillover affected sleep and appetite and, as seems almost inevitably to occur in chronically painful states, the opposite half of the body. Whimsical perhaps, but just as adjacent gyroscopes will harmonize with each other, so will the different halves of the brain. The ability of the subcortical brain to isolate left from right is quite limited. In a sense, unilateral chronic pain is quite as unnatural as unilateral depression or unilateral schizophrenia.

When acute pain becomes chronic, it crosses the midline. Fibromyalgia and chronic headache are almost never unilateral. In those diseases, the dissemination of pain from one body part to another we have tended to ascribe to imagination or depression, or to some sort of unempowerment. We are unable to do that with reflex sympathetic dystrophy. The phenomenon is so visible and so organic that we simply have to recognize it as the capacity of a plastic brain to reconfigure.

I will digress briefly from Luz's story to describe another patient who illustrates the incredible capacity of chronic pain to move one body part to another. She awoke one morning with a sensation of burning in her mucosal surfaces—her mouth, vagina, and rectum. Her pain began in central structures, right down the middle. It appeared during a stressful interval when her husband was incapacitated with cancer. She became sleep-disordered, fatigued, and depressed. She consulted many physicians, some in faraway referral centers. Her treatments included cortisone and immunosuppressants for a presumed neuritic pain, perhaps due to lupus. They were totally without effect.

I listened to her story with great credulity. I had seen enough painful patients and heard enough bizarre descriptions of the placements of pain to accept their descriptions unreservedly and without judgment. As I treated her and she began to improve, her pain abandoned mucosal surfaces and migrated laterally, into her cutaneous ones, her face and torso. Along the way I made several drug adjustments. When they were ineffective and her pain worsened, it would move back to the mucosal surface. With favorable treatment, it moved back into the skin. I watched, over the course of several months, a brain under the influence of pharmacotherapy playing ping-pong with itself. As she finally improved, erratically and very slowly, her midline mucosal pain diminished first and only later, her more lateral. Months into her treatment she reported to me that the skin of her arms and legs was beginning to burn. When she told me this, I knew I was winning the game. In the end her pain went slowly away, discharging itself through the digits, the tips of her fingers and toes. It is quite impossible to explain this lady's experience on the basis of a disease of peripheral nerves. We would have to recruit a disorder of millions of cells widely scattered throughout the body. In the brain, however, a change in the focus of neuronal activity of only a few millimeters would easily account for the dissemination of painfulness. The pain is in the brain, and it can shift from place to place, it seems, with astonishing ease.

Luz and I ultimately developed a good relationship, but at first it was difficult. She carried great bitterness and suspicion, perhaps rightly so. Her physicians, after all, had failed her badly. I was not to blame. All the procedures and all the torment had occurred before she came to me. All I could do was pick up the pieces.

There were, thank God, no more operations available to Luz. I maintained her opiate therapy and treated her with tricyclics and many other drugs. They helped her sleep, but only a little. It was probably naïve to expect much improvement. Too much time had passed. Luz and I settled down for the long haul, and I considered my treatment choices. They were few.

There was one treatment modality left, but it is better in theory than in practice (as were most of the operations performed on Luz). When we use mind drugs for pain we are attempting to restore to function unused analgesic systems. In the face of ongoing opiate therapy, however, these systems become atrophic, in much the same manner that the thyroid and adrenal glands cease functioning when they are placed at rest by the administration of thyroid or cortisone. Removing the painful from opiate therapy plausibly will restore, with the aid of drugs such as the tricyclics, dormant brain centers into effective functioning. Denying opiate therapy to the painful patient seems counterintuitive and perhaps cruel. The treatment form is, as I have said, better in theory than in practice. Still, many— probably most—patients on long-term opiate therapy could get by without it. In Luz's case, it was worth a try. Her opiates were a burden, a medical, financial, and social burden. She was admitted to the hospital, and with the assistance of an addictionologist, I attempted to withdraw her from Demerol. As with every other intervention with Luz, it was an absolute failure. With each incre- mental reduction in drug dosage, her pain and her behaviors worsened. I may have suffered a disorder of imagination as I observed her. Her stump actually seemed to get colder as we reduced her opiates! The addictionologist concluded that it was quite unrealistic to deprive this woman of opiate therapy. With that it was written in stone. Luz would remain on opiates, probably for the rest of her life.

I watched, over the course of several months, a brain under the influence of pharmacotherapy playing ping-pong with itself.

I tried several opiates, a slow-release preparation of oral morphine known as MS Contin, and later Duragesic, a drug adminis- tered transcutaneously through a patch applied to the skin. These delivery systems are desirable because there are no peaks and troughs in blood levels. A steady state and hopefully more even analgesia can be obtained. Luz tolerated neither. I knew I had to discard Demerol. With prolonged high dosage use, it can produce seizures. I was left with Dilaudid. Perhaps the strongest and most addictive opioid, it was also the one with the most street value.

I gave Luz staggering quantities of Dilaudid, and I gave her something else. I gave her trust. That, I think, was quite as important in her care as her opiate therapy. Luz had been shuttled from doctor to doctor. Her various operations were performed at major medical centers throughout the eastern half of the nation. When she found me she at least had, for better or worse, one doctor and for the first time a predictable, regular pattern of care. I did not harangue Luz about her use of the drugs. I provided them with measured care.

Some physicians use opiates comfortably and fearlessly and ascribe great benefit to them. I suspect that their success relates to more than just the analgesic effect of opiates. It is the predictability of the drugs' availability and the freedom from suspicion and guilt that really helps. This belief does not represent a mere abstraction. Just as children find their way to behavioral health through the rightful assembly of neural configurations in an environment of regularity, predictability, nurture, and trust, so do painful patients find their way to recovery.

Luz gradually got better. Painfulness often improves with time. Just why this happens is uncertain. It may relate to some form of cerebral exhaustion. Maladaptive behaviors are energy inefficient and wasteful and, therefore, unsustainable. Spontaneous recovery from depression, schizophrenia, and painfulness does occur, probably because wellness is more efficient than illness.

Luz seemed to be compliant with her drug therapy, never coming by for early refills. There were none of the usual fabrications. No stolen drugs, no shorting of prescriptions, no flush-down-the-toilet accidents. I never identified the slurred speech and clumsiness of drug intoxication, although I looked closely for them. I watched Luz slowly improve, this over a couple of years. Her painful behaviors diminished. Even her hyperpathia began to dissipate. I was witness to a slow miracle. I suspected it was a function of time and not her opiate therapy.

I could usually, but not always, find the presence of Dilaudid in Luz's blood and urine. I could never find the other drugs I was administering. Luz was not as compliant as I had thought. She was taking the drugs of her choice, not mine. I continued to provide Dilaudid, and I never betrayed my suspicions as I watched my patient month after month get better. She remained sleepless and appetite-deprived, but her angst was abating. Her pain had become, as chronic pain usually does, a partner rather than an intruder. Opiate therapy, so valuable early on, had become, with time, more or less irrelevant. Her medicine, I suspected, was becoming more useful sold than swallowed. Again, the conundrum of opiate therapy. Drugs prescribed by compassionate and well-meaning physicians often end up in the hands of people who use them for recreation. Sad to say, chronic pain can be, for the victim, a very profitable illness.

I did not want to punish Luz. That's not by job. God knows, she had been punished enough. The physician must remove himself from judgment and anger. They have no place in the care of a patient, but sometimes they are unavoidable emotions. I pondered Luz's care for quite a long time. My clinical decisions had to be removed from anger at what I perceived to be her deceit. I did not threaten her with my suspicions. That would serve no purpose. I decided, however, that it was time once again to attempt withdrawal from opiates. Years had passed, and Luz was better. Her improvement had occurred, not through the agency of my skills or her opiate therapy, but through the agency of time. I advised Luz, indeed I gave her no choice, that we were going to attempt detox again. For the first time in her unfortunate painful existence, something worked. She was withdrawn from her opiates without difficulty. Her pain and sleeplessness actually diminished.

Where she is now and what she is doing I know not, but I think of her often. What turns has her life taken? A young woman now in her thirties, her cerebral matrix possessed of incredible experiences, of pain, of amputation, of penetration with electrodes and cautery, and years of opiate use. Will any of these be resurrected along the way as she meets untoward life events and circumstances? We can only wonder.

Christy was scheduled for cystoscopy. This procedure is performed under light intravenous anesthesia to visualize the urinary bladder. Christy's nurse had difficulty finding a vein for intravenous access. Repeated attempts to place a needle in the forearm were unsuccessful and Christy, over the course of a half-hour, was punctured several times. She became quite angry. The nurse, frustrated also, attempted once again to enter a vein, this time in the wrist. She struck the median nerve with the needle, and Christy immediately experienced severe pain in her hand. Minor nerve trauma due to inadvertent placement of intravenous needles is not rare. The initial experience is quite painful, but it usually goes away very quickly when the needle is withdrawn. That didn't happen in Christy. Her pain, already kindled by repeated passes in the arm, didn't go away. The procedure was terminated, but the damage had been done. Christy was on her way to reflex sympathetic dystrophy.

Her hand was painful, cold, sweaty, and hyperpathic. An anesthesiologist performed a sympathetic block. The hand warmed and dried, but there was no relief from pain. Clearly that treatment modality was going nowhere. Her physicians debated the merits of surgically exploring the carpal tunnel to see if the median nerve had become scarred or entrapped. The surgery made sense, but they were uneasy. Median nerve injuries due to the carpal tunnel syndrome are a dime a dozen, but they almost never produce the florid autonomic response that Christy exhibited.

For most of her adult life Christy had been painful and depressed. She had a family history of migraine, and she suffered that disease with attacks of great frequency. Early on, when she was in her twenties, her headaches responded to the drug Imitrex, but later when they became almost incessant, they no longer responded. She suffered interstitial cystitis with chronic pelvic discomfort and frequent painful voidings. This was the reason for her cystoscopy. She had used many drugs for her depression. Prozac was the best, but even its benefits were incomplete. She was sleepless and subject to frequent awakenings. Along the way she developed a weight gain problem, some fifty pounds over three years. She complained of severe fatigue and reported that her memory was becoming impaired, a problem for her as an accountant.

I composed my letter to Christy's physicians with care. There certainly had been a median nerve injury, but this had occurred in a premorbid state of sleeplessness, fatigue, chronic cystitis, headache, depression, and perhaps importantly, by anger. I concurred with the decision to explore the median nerve but suggested that we wait a bit, that we undertake a trial of drug therapy before jumping into surgery. If we could simply restore her diurnal rhythms, allow her to sleep, and perhaps improve her depression and fatigue, she would be a much better operative candidate than if we had not.

I cautioned against the use of opiates (Christy had been on Darvon and Hydrocodone without much benefit). I forbade their usage and prescribed Imipramine and Klonopin. After several days her sleep improved. There was a little morning sedation, not uncommon with the drugs, but there was also a sense of refreshment and restoration, something Christy had not known throughout her adult life. Her hand pain continued about as before but, remarkably, her headaches remitted. Formerly incessant, they became only occasional, and when they did occur they responded, once again, to Imitrex. Her pelvic pain diminished also, and the uncomfortable voidings became less frequent. I reintroduced Neurontin, a drug of known effectiveness in the treatment of pain. It had been tried before without success, but for that matter so had Imitrex. The effect of a drug, it bears emphasis, often changes according to time and circumstance. Neurontin on top of Imipramine and Klonopin helped. Neurontin alone had not. Christy's hand pain diminished significantly. I was employing polypharmacy. It wasn't symptomatic treatment. It wasn't rational treatment. It was empiric treatment, based simply on the knowledge that there is usually a drug out there that will work.

Christy was sleep-restored and mood-stabilized. She was ready for her operation. The nerve was explored and released from pressure within a scarred carpal tunnel. Her hand pain dissipated, at least partially, and her life became more agreeable. Free of headaches, bladder pain, fatigue, and insomnia, she also experienced a delightful bonus. Her appetite diminished and she began to lose weight.

I was thrilled with the outcome. No cure perhaps, but close to it. Christy could have easily gone the way of Luz. One operation after another, one failure-to-recover after another. It didn't happen though, and I suspect it was because I was able to employ drug therapy not only for her reflex sympathetic dystrophy but also the underlying depression that anticipated it. What would have happened with Luz if the drugs had gotten in early, before her tragedy evolved?

CHAPTER TWELVE

Kindling

A young woman goes away to college. It is an experience of delight and discovery for her, but also one of stress. Academic and social pressures overwhelm, and a mind, formerly resourceful and elastic, is bent. She enters a depressive interlude. She may experience tearful despondency, or perhaps a syndrome of fatigue, apathy, and disinterest. Regardless, she will likely recover spontaneously. First depressions usually do. Later in her young life she encounters another stressor, a parental divorce. Depression comes quicker and deeper this time. Spontaneous recovery is less certain, but even so, with time and perhaps drug therapy, her depression abates, and she enters an interval of wellness. Her disease, however, is now ingrained and subject to recrudescence. Throughout the remainder of her life this woman will experience interludes of depression, sometimes in response to a stressful provocation, but often in the absence of any identifiable stressor. An alternate behavior is established, and recurrent depression appears randomly through her life.

Many diseases exhibit this natural history. They appear initially under provocation. At their onset they are stimulus-dependent. Epilepsy in the child, for instance, may be precipitated by flickering lights, and migraine by a host of stressors which we identify as triggers. Migraine, epilepsy, and depression are all recurrent diseases. They reappear under provocation. With each recurrence, the neural systems subserving them become more integrated and fixed. They become, if you will, more confident and sure of themselves. Ultimately they acquire a life of their own.

They begin to appear even in the absence of provocation. They become stimulus-independent. This is the phenomenon of *kindling*. Neural systems, by dint of repetition, incite alternate behaviors which recur throughout life.

The kindling theory is a widely accepted and convenient explanation for the recurrent nature of many neuropsychiatric illnesses. Aggressive treatment of epilepsy, migraine, and depression is warranted, not only for the sake of patient comfort, but to prevent kindling, that is to prevent the later recurrence of the disorder. Painfulness, certainly as much a cerebral experience as epilepsy and depression, may also be kindled.

Remember Helen, gang-raped as a teenager. Following that event, her menstrual cramping worsened. Her pain was, at least initially, stimulus-dependent. With each succeeding menstruation, the neural processing of pain was kindled and ultimately it became incessant and stimulus-independent. Her chronic pelvic pain was ascribed to endometriosis, but the definitive treatment of that disorder did not relieve her. It simply transferred the pain, by a process of referral, to her back. Her physicians thought she had lumbar disc disease. You know the rest of the story.

Lumbar disc disease is often a recurrent and progressive disorder. One disc after another ruptures, and in the process vertebral alignment is disordered. Spinal instability ensues, and as the disease advances, arthritis and the constriction of nerves by scar tissue gradually develops. Pain evolves from a relatively simple mechanical disorder, an extruded disc impinging on a nerve, to a much more complex and confusing illness. It is hard to make generalizations about a disease as complicated as the failed back, but there is one that I believe will stand even the most critical analysis. That is, as the disease progresses, the precise pain generator becomes less easy to identify. The longer the disease lasts, the less certain we are of its true nature. This is, I suspect, because of kindling.

David was an electrician. As a young man, about age thirty-five, he experienced a ruptured lumbar disc with sciatica. Surgery was performed, and he was cured. Free of pain, he continued to work effectively and productively for many years until an adjacent disc ruptured. He suffered another interval of back and leg pain and required a second operation. This too was successful, although it took David a bit longer to recover. Years later his sciatica recurred. Imaging studies demonstrated no certain disc protrusion, but there was some vertebral instability, plausibly the pain generator. The orthopedist suggested a lumbar fusion. Prospects for success were good, he thought. After all, David had responded rather well to his previous surgeries. An operation was performed but with little benefit. David remained painful, and he became sleepless and depressed. The surgeon prescribed Triavil. It was recognized in that era as a drug that was good for both pain and depression. David improved and was able to go back to work. I doubt that the orthopedist was aware in any degree that he was treating a kindled behavior. He was simply using a convenient drug for insomnia, depression, and pain. It was the drug, not the surgery, that helped David.

A state of pain is a cerebral as well as corporal experience, and these two cannot be separated. That which happens to the body happens without exception also to the mind.

Then a stroke of bad luck. David had a routine physical examination, and his internist, discovering his use of Triavil, told him to discard it. It was a dangerous agent, capable of producing dyskinesia. A few weeks later, the requisite few weeks, David's pain reappeared in his back and both legs, and he re-entered a depression. A kindled behavior, free of pharmacologic restraint, was becoming operational. The well-meaning internist prescribed Prozac for depression and referred David once again to the orthopedist. Imaging studies this time were negative. There was no certain accountant for the recurrent pain. The fusion seemed to be in good order, but sometimes a broken fusion cannot be seen on imaging studies, and the surgeon elected to perform an exploratory operation. He must have congratulated himself when he discovered that one of the bony fusions had indeed broken down. It was fused again, this time with metallic hardware to support the vertebrae. David didn't get any better at all. (You can't cure kindled behavior with hardware.) His postoperative imaging studies showed good vertebral alignment and stability and no evidence of nerve compression, but David remained incessantly painful and progressively depressed. His pain, which had been stimulus-dependent, sciatica due to a ruptured disc, had become stimulus-independent, the failed back.

David found his way to me, and recounted his medical history. The sequential development of his painfulness was clearly evident. I told him to resume the Triavil, and he got better, substantially better. He did not get well, however. It was too late for that. David, at age fifty-seven, had to retire.

The kindling theory is a simple conceptual and organizational idea. It makes common sense, and it can be transcribed into many illness behaviors. Substance abuse begins as stimulus-dependent behavior— alcohol for the relief of anxiety or insomnia, opiates for the relief of pain. Both later become stimulus-independent. Post-traumatic stress disorder begins as stimulus dependent, but the behaviors continue after the stimulus has been removed. Epilepsy, migraine, depression, substance abuse, post-traumatic stress disorder, and painfulness all obey the same natural history.

We really should recognize that the phenomenon of kindling is operative in chronic pain as it is in so many other illnesses. There is a barrier, however, and that is the mind-body dichotomy. "This pain can't be in my mind. This pain is real!" These two declamations are, of course, not mutually exclusive. The pain is real, and it is in the mind. A state of pain is a cerebral as well as corporal experience, and these two cannot be separated. That which happens to the body happens without exception also to the mind.

As a young man George was damaged badly in an automobile accident. He was blinded, and both lower extremities amputated. He survived the ordeal, married, and found employment as a police dispatcher. Throughout his life he experienced phantom limb pain, not unexpected after a violent amputation incurred in youth. He cohabited with the experience. It was random, erratic, and usually brief. He never sought medical attention for it until about age sixty when his phantom pain became, over the course of a few weeks, more severe. He consulted his physician and was treated with the tricyclic Doxepin. George's pain diminished. Why this worsening of his pain should have happened so remote in time from the original experience was, I believe, never pursued. No need, perhaps. He got better with drug therapy and that was that.

George's disordered brain was not to be easily intimidated by drug therapy. He had another painful experience. He passed a kidney stone. He had suffered them occasionally throughout his life, a half dozen times or so. Following his last kidney stone attack, however, George's pain didn't quite go away. It wasn't severe, but it did linger. A few weeks later he developed another kidney stone. This one impacted and would not pass. An operation for its removal was performed successfully, but George's pain did not abate. He became progressively sleepless and fatigued. In this setting, as we could certainly predict, his phantom limb pain recurred, more extravagantly than ever before. I assumed his care and reviewed his history, knowing that this sequence of events could not simply have appeared out of the blue. Surely something had happened to this man to account for the fact that his recurrent pains, certainly kindled but nonetheless restrained for so many years, had late in his life become operative, unfolding into relentless pain.

George was a highly controlled person, not given to emotion. I searched for antecedents for his late life onset painfulness. He denied drug or alcohol use. There had been no prior history of depression. George described his life as one of order and regularity, and he denied any intercurrent emotional stress. As I continued my interrogations, inquiring about his home and his relationships, he remarked that he and his wife had recently divorced. It was, he said, by mutual agreement. After forty years, they had separated amicably and without disharmony. George discounted the significance of the event. He was, he said, in no way distressed. Not so. George's wife left him for a younger man, and George—his

protestations notwithstanding—was clearly altered by the experience. It all had to come out some way. It could have been and
perhaps should have been depression, but George, throughout his
remarkable life, had never known that experience. He had,
however, known pain. Those memories, kindled over the years,
found expression under the provocation of a life event. It reads so
clearly if we simply take time to search the history.

Blinded and amputated though George was, he had a
profoundly healthy neurobiology. His infrastructure was intact.
The dominant behavior of wellness in the face of adversity had
been extant throughout his life. Recruiting it was a simple matter, if
we can call the capacity of pharmaceuticals to reroute cerebral
activity simple. I administered Klonopin and increased dosages of
Doxepin, a drug which had already demonstrated its effectiveness,
and George got well. His pain, even his phantom limb, went away.
George's pains, limb and renal, had been kindled by repetition
throughout his life. In wellness their display was arrested until the
termination of a marriage allowed their escape. Experiential memories found expression.

The mature patient with recent onset pain usually responds very
well to psychopharmaceuticals. This is somewhat contrary to what
we would expect. We could reasonably anticipate that the young,
capacious, and resourceful brain would be more responsive to drug
therapy than the less plastic brain of the older person. By no means
does it always happen this way. The mature brain has assembled a
host of integrated and adaptive systems. There is a lot to fall back
on. It is the integrity of this infrastructure that dictates response to
drugs quite as much as their pharmacologic effect. We cannot now,
nor will we in the foreseeable future fully comprehend how and
why drugs make painful patients better. For the time being we must
simply ascribe their efficacy to their remarkable capacity to reconfigure the reconfiguration—to restore discarded systems and
behaviors back into function. This is the reason why pharmacotherapy is so ineffective in the treatment of pain and maladaptive
behaviors which attend early childhood sexual abuse. There is no

infrastructure, and without it there is limited capacity to respond to drug therapy. This is why autism, infantile schizophrenia, is so unresponsive to pharmacotherapy. There is no infrastructure at all. Nothing to fall back on. No wellness behaviors to recruit.

CHAPTER THIRTEEN

Substance Abuse

The most commonly used drug is ethyl alcohol. It produces a pleasant sense of relaxation and disinhibition, this we believe by stimulating GABA receptors. Used in moderation, it probably has no long-term adverse effects. In excess it is toxic to neural tissue. This may manifest as peripheral neuritis with numbness, tingling, and sometimes pain in the extremities. Less common is cerebellar degeneration with ataxia due to destruction of the brain's balance center. Occasionally a portion of the limbic system may be selectively destroyed, producing memory loss, alcoholic dementia.

Alcohol is a drug of abuse, and it has the capacity in those perhaps genetically predisposed to produce addiction. Abstinence from the drug in those dependent upon it will invoke withdrawal, tremors, convulsive seizures, or delirium tremens. There is another withdrawal effect, not so widely recognized, and that is painfulness. It usually appears within a short interval following alcohol withdrawal, a few weeks or months, but it may occur years later. This is not unlike the occurrence of delirium tremens. That disorder typically comes within a week or two of withdrawal, but in exceptional cases it may appear many years later just as it did with Harry. In his case delirium tremens occurred in time remote from his alcohol withdrawal under the provocation of a stressor, carcinoma of the esophagus.

The resiliency and redundancy of our neural systems allow us, most of the time, to compensate and override potentially maladaptive behaviors. This is quite evident in alcoholism. Most can enter abstinence without major withdrawal. However, if there is an intercurrent stressor such as pneumonia or hip fracture, delirium tremens occurs with great predictability. A combination of stressors overwhelms the body's capacity for defense. This may account for the occurrence of painfulness after alcohol withdrawal. There are often concurrent stressors, sometimes depression and sometimes corporal injury from which the patient fails to recover.

Joe's young life had been dominated by risk-seeking, violence, and alcoholism. His credits included DUIs, motorcycle accidents, and twenty-four hours of coma from a concussion sustained in a barroom altercation. Joe never did anything halfway. His social and personal behaviors knew no restraint. Predictably, when he fell in love, that experience was also unrestrained. His passion for his motorcycle and his drink was replaced by that for his woman and her church. He discovered religion, married, and renounced his habit. Within a couple of months he became fibromyalgia-painful in his neck, shoulders, and back. In the course of his treatment he was given Naprosyn, an anti-inflammatory drug commonly used for musculoskeletal pain. He suffered a side effect in the form of enterocolitis. His diarrhea persisted even after cessation of Naprosyn. During the course of his evaluation, he underwent colonoscopy and suffered an inadvertent blowout of his colon. Emergency surgery was necessary to repair the leak. Joe failed to recover. He became chronically abdomen-painful even though his anatomy was restored and his diarrhea cured.

The syndrome of the irresponsible alcoholic youth entering recovery and painfulness should be better recognized. It is a common clinical occurrence. Joe came to me pretty early in the game, just a few months from the onset of his symptoms. He responded brilliantly to Nortriptyline and Klonopin. This may have been because his brain was young and reactive and capable of response, but I think the real reason was that I got to him quickly. His disease had not had time to become kindled beyond repair.

Rex had been alcoholic in his youth with several incarcerations, including a stay in prison for attempted murder. That experience got his attention, and he entered abstinence. In a short while he became back painful. A ruptured lumbar disc was identified and surgery was done, but his pain continued. He was treated with the analgesic Darvon. The drug was reasonably effective, and he continued to work for many years as a truck driver, taking eight to ten capsules daily. What Rex did, of course, was to substitute Darvon dependency for alcohol dependency. An irresponsible behavior was replaced by a more responsible one, the treatment of pain. Another syndrome—the recovered alcoholic, painful and on drugs of abuse, regularly attending AA meetings.

I saw Rex many years into his illness. I did not get to him quickly, and I had no luck at all. His alcohol-induced painfulness had been kindled over many years, and the prospect of neural reconfiguration and healing was prohibited by his ongoing use of a substance of abuse. The only way that Rex could get well, and there is no guarantee at all that this would happen because of the long duration of his illness, would be withdrawal from his Darvon and the institution of more appropriate pharmacy. Rex could not countenance this prospect. He was drug-dependent, and this behavior extended over decades—first alcohol and then Darvon. Rex thanked me for my efforts but said, "You know, Doc, these Darvons are the only thing that have ever given me any relief."

Rachel came to see me for her pelvic pain. She was recently discharged from a faraway treatment center which she had entered a month before for yet another attempt at cure of her polysubstance abuse. She had used marijuana, cocaine, and alcohol for many years, and she had been through detox several times. After each treatment, she would enter a few months of sobriety and then relapse back into her disease. This last attempt, a month inpatient stay at a major center, was going to be her best shot. It had gone especially well this time. Rachel was proud of her progress and so were her counselors. Her prognosis, they felt, was excellent. Just a little fly in the ointment though. Late in her stay Rachel developed pelvic discomfort and painful voiding. A simple urinary tract infection, it seemed. Antibiotics were prescribed. A follow-up urinalysis was normal, but her pain continued. Nonetheless, she was discharged and advised to seek the attention of a physician in her community. Her counselors should have known better.

She was in her mid-thirties, somewhat obese, and animated and obsessive about her painfulness, which was worsening by the day. I reviewed her history anticipating it would be pregnant with meaning. Rachel told me that both of her parents were alcoholic, and she acknowledged childhood physical abuse. Rachel had received, as many like her have, a double hit.

She had experienced attacks of pelvic pain along the way and also depression and sleeplessness. She could temper these symptoms for a while with drugs of abuse. When they failed, as they always did, she would enter recovery at a treatment center. Wellness could never be sustained, however, and she would again become sympto-matic with depression, sleeplessness, and pelvic pain.

As Rachel and I discussed our treatment choices, we encoun-tered a common clinical conundrum. She had entered wellness through the cessation of drugs of abuse. Her continued recovery was predicated, she was sure, on abstinence from any and all such agents. She looked with disfavor on my recommendation that she begin pharmacy with, among other drugs, benzodiazepines, poten-tially addictive agents.

I don't know the answer to this problem. Rachel might have responded to drug therapy. It wouldn't have been easy, for sure, but there was at least some prospect for improvement. This would, of course, entail the use of some of the very agents she had been taught to avoid. Introduction of these drugs would carry risk for the resumption of her addictive behaviors. Without them, however, her pain would only worsen. Rachel and I deliberated together, and she chose to sustain her recovery, painful though it was.

James was a heavy equipment mechanic. Perhaps because of the exertions and traumas imposed by that trade he developed cervical spondylosis, with disc and vertebral degeneration sufficient to compress the spinal cord and nerve roots. He suffered pain in his arms and hands and progressive weakness in his lower extremities. Cervical decompression was done. The vertebral column was unroofed, relieving pressure on the spinal cord, and the neural foramina were opened, allowing more space for the nerve roots. His leg weakness improved following surgery, but James's hand pain worsened. It was more severe after surgery than before. Imaging studies demonstrated no cause.

James's father died young, and he and his brother were raised in the projects. He experimented with drugs of abuse, first alcohol through his teen years and later amphetamines. Then came marijuana and finally cocaine. He used it regularly for many years. James then entered a sort of spontaneous recovery, but it was incomplete. He continued to use alcohol and not infrequently marijuana, but the quantity was much diminished. The fates, it seems, should have rewarded James better than they did, but it was not to be so. When James developed nociceptive (pain-generating) pathology in the form of cervical spondylosis, his analgesic system, physiologically withered by years of drug abuse, was incapable of responding. His pain was only in part the product of nerve damage. It was equally the product of substance abuse.

It is not surprising at all that this syndrome of disordered sleep is so frequently associated with painfulness.

Bill was referred by a neurologist of great competence. He was in his seventies, a retired businessman. He lived in the fast lane and made lots of money. He also drank a lot, but it had never been a real problem. No DUIs, no accidents. "I was lucky," said Bill. His alcohol consumption extended over many years, but on the date of his wife's death from lung cancer, he renounced his whiskey and his cigarettes and entered a life of despondency.

He was jowly, thick-necked, and obese, the typical habitus of the patient with sleep apnea. It is not surprising at all that this syndrome of disordered sleep is so frequently associated with painfulness. By virtue of carrying too much weight in the tissues of the neck and throat, the patient with sleep apnea suffers an upper airway obstruction. During sleep, the fatty pharynx and neck collapse into the airway, and the victim, sucking air into his lungs against an obstruction, snores loudly. After an interval of progressive snoring, which simply represents labored respiratory effort, exhaustion supervenes, and respiration stops. Blood oxygen tension falls to a critical level, and this is a stimulant for the somnolent brain to awaken and start breathing again. During these apneic, anoxic intervals, sleep is interrupted, and effective and restorative patterns of sleep are never achieved. Daytime somnolence and fatigue are hallmarks of the heavy snorer, as is painfulness. Bill was treated with a continuous positive airway pressure (CPAP) device, a mask which provides increased pressure to overcome airway resistance, and he found it helpful. He also found it, as most patients using the device do, to be somewhat inconvenient. Bill's life, one of loneliness and depression, was already inconvenienced enough. He was an accident waiting to happen.

He began to experience sharp painful electric sensations throughout his body. These were brief and lancinating, not sustained at first. They had a curious predilection for appearing in his testicles and eyes. Near midline structures all, the four roundest things in his body became painful. Why, we can only guess. Some sort of symbol perhaps. Maybe a reflection of a latent phobia. Most of us, after all, are somewhat fearful of their loss.

Bill's pain continued to affect his round things, but less so. It gradually became predominant in, of all places, his toes. They were constantly burning and painful. This certainly suggested an alcoholic neuritis, but his tactile and vibratory sensations were normal, and nerve conduction studies showed no evidence of neuritis. Bill's pain was not coming from his feet. It was coming from his mind.

CPAP notwithstanding, Bill's sleep was nonrestorative. No longer disturbed by apneic awakenings, it was interrupted by pain in his toes, which awoke him repetitively through the night. He was depressed, but he had not responded in any meaningful way to an SSRI administered by his neurologist. He was thought-disordered, obsessing about his pain. It was quite impossible to converse with him about any issue other than his painfulness.

Bill's physical examination was well recorded by the neurologist. He had a low amplitude, rather fast tremor in his hands. This was recognized as an *essential* tremor, a benign, nonthreatening, but inconveniencing and embarrassing hand movement. It had been treated with limited success with the drug Mysoline. Curiously, as Bill became painful, his hand tremor diminished. He experienced improvement in one illness simultaneously with worsening of another. No need to belabor why this should happen. It probably represented a form of cerebral exhaustion, the inability to sustain multiple maladaptive behaviors simultaneously. Regardless, he still had a little hand tremor when I saw him, and it was a bit confusing because, as I watched and examined Bill, observing his painful toes, they exhibited a tremor quite unlike that in his hands. There was no oscillation, no to-and-fro movement. Rather, each toe would move in turn, one after the other, at a frequency of about two per second. A most unusual movement, a toe-tap tremor, it was quite different from that in his hands.

Tremors are common and sometimes confusing disorders. Most of them were described a century or so ago, and bear Greek-derived identifiers such as dystonia, dyskinesia, and myoclonus. Other tremors, those identified in more recent times, have been accorded a more prosaic nomenclature. Essential tremor is certainly a pedestrian use of words, and so is restless legs. Nonetheless, it is a rather good descriptor, for it identifies the disorder for what it is, a sensation of being unable to hold the legs still. In a sense, the tremor has been trivialized by its descriptive name. Nonetheless, it is an important and common movement disorder. In most cases it is generated by attempts to sleep, and it is very common in people with chronic pain. It also occurs with great frequency in alcoholics, usually those who have entered recovery. Certainly another manifestation of withdrawal.

I was quite surprised when Bill responded to my question that he had never experienced anything like restless legs. With his history of alcoholism and his painfulness, I would have predicted with great certainty that he suffered this tremor. As I was about to conclude that he was just a rare alcoholic, painful bird without restless legs, it dawned on me that he was not unafflicted. He didn't have restless legs, but he did have restless toes, a *forme fruste* perhaps.

The association of this particular movement disorder with painfulness is being increasingly recognized.

Painfulness and movement disorder. Painfulness and depression. Painfulness and obsessions. Painfulness and disordered sleep and appetite and energy. Painfulness and substance abuse. All reflect the interactivity of disordered analgesic systems with other subcortical functions. Chronic pain is a disease of cerebral disharmony, expressing itself in myriad ways.

Bill did very well with Klonopin, Imipramine, and Neurontin. His sleep returned and his pain went away. Depression cleared and the tremors, in both hands and toes, diminished. As often happens in the treatment of the painful, when the right drugs kick in, everything gets better.

Our toes are that part of us most far from the brain. Sensory axons transmitting their message have further to travel than those from any other body part. They are longer and, therefore, more susceptible to injury. Not only are they most far from the brain, they are also most far from the heart. Their blood supply is the least of any other body part. This is probably the reason why alcoholic neuritis appears so typically and almost exclusively in the toes and not in the fingers. Bill, however, suffered no neuritis. His was a central pain syndrome. Originating in the brain, it expressed itself through the toes. Why did disordered nature in the endgame pick on the toes? We can only speculate.

Bill's pain began in the most richly sensory innervated structures in the body, the eyes and the testicles. These are also organs greatly endowed with symbolic value. As Bill's brain struggled to overcome his disorder, those organs most rich in neural and symbolic authority fell under the dominance of a brain trying to right itself. But the righting, as is often the case, was incomplete. In the end, Bill experienced his pain in his toes, that part most distal and under the least sway of central authority.

CHAPTER FOURTEEN

Bipolarity

The bipolar patient experiences times of wellness and emotional equilibrium alternating with intervals of depression and others of manic hyperactivity. With these swings in mood and behavior, the entire neural axis reconfigures and exhibits almost unbelievable effects. Some bipolars suffer tremors, even dyskinesia, during depressive interludes with total disappearance of these during mania. A change in dominant handedness may occur: left-handed when depressed, right-handed when manic! In a notable case reported many years ago, a bipolar patient was conversant only in the Gaelic language when he was depressed. During mania, he became fluent only in the English language! In another case, even more remarkable, a brain-damaged, hemiplegic, and aphasic patient experienced the restoration of speech and movement during manic intervals. If bipolar disease can do these things, what can it not do?

Henry was a mechanic. He retired on account of chronic back pain incurred in an automobile accident in which he suffered a compression fracture and a ruptured lumbar disc. He came to surgery, and his spine was fused. Vertebral alignment was stabilized, but Henry remained painful and unable to work. Most of the time his discomfort was tolerable and responsive to low-grade analgesics, but occasionally he experienced sudden sieges of excruciating pain. A reasonably effective treatment form evolved. During the attacks his orthopedist would admit him to the hospital and treat him with intravenous opiates and muscle relaxants. After a few days—the sieges were all rather brief—Henry would settle down, go home, and resume with only modest inconvenience his sedentary life. This pattern extended over more than a decade with a hospital admission once or twice a year. Henry's orthopedist, a very wise man, recognized this as a very unusual behavior. Chronic pain due to an injured back is certainly well-known to orthopedists, but the intermittency of Henry's attacks was very queer.

Henry resisted referral to me. He was doing just fine, he said, on this treatment program and was quite happy with it. His attacks were always short-lived and opiate-responsive. Gradually, however, they became more frequent, and he finally accepted my consultation.

When the doctor hears the phrase, "everything is better now," it usually means that the doctor is treating the very core of the disease.

Henry was not a very charming man, laconic and a bit on the gruff side. I saw him during an interval of relative wellness, and I couldn't find much to work with. His behaviors were quite unremarkable. His sleep was slightly disturbed, appropriate to his painfulness, but it was not a major handicap, and Henry evidenced no depression. I knew there was something odd about this, but it seemed reasonable to begin therapy with a tricyclic, hopefully to abort future attacks of pain. Several weeks into his treatment, Henry called me complaining of another attack of back pain. He requested hospitalization and opiate treatment and demanded that the orthopedist, to whom he was very attached, remain in attendance. I arranged the admission and began the treatment protocol which had been initiated by his surgeon. I hoped to uncover some clues during his hospitalization. I certainly had found none thus far. Henry was quite uncomfortable and back-stiffened, but there was otherwise no change in his neurologic status, nor was there any discernible change in behavior. He was neither restless nor despondent. Henry seemed to be pretty much the same man when he was painful as when he was not.

After a week in the hospital during which, with opiates, he achieved a high degree of comfort, he declared that he was ready to go home. I discontinued the tricyclic therapy. On his return, Henry was his usual opinionated self. He told me that this siege had been like all the rest, sudden severe upper lumbar back pain without radiation. He emphasized again that his opiate therapy was profoundly helpful to him, and he would not countenance being denied that treatment when his severe pain recurred.

I couldn't figure Henry out. Opiate-responsive pain, nothing startling there, but a cyclical opiate-responsive pain. This was certainly not addictive behavior. After a short course of opiates he had no further need. He received them on an intermittent, never a regular basis. I chose Lithium. A long shot maybe, but the strange periodicity of his pain merited attention. The drug is reasonably safe in low dosage and a convenient agent for therapeutic trial. I instructed Henry that if the drug disagreed with him to simply discard it, but if he felt any benefit at all to continue taking three hundred milligrams of it each night.

I saw him a month later, and he did seem different. Usually dour, he exhibited more spontaneity. There was a twinkle in his eye, and Henry was not a person in whom you would expect a twinkle.

"I like that Lithium."

"What do you mean you like Lithium?"

"I just feel different. Everything is better now."

"Is your pain any better?"

"Yes, sort of, I guess. It's still there, but it doesn't bother me the way it used to."

Often in the treatment of pain the physician finds the absolutely perfect drug. I had seen it many times with Triavil and on other occasions with tricyclics and benzodiazepines. This time it was Lithium. When the right drug kicks in, there is a sense, sometimes immediately, that *everything is better*. I had elected to use Lithium simply on the basis of the periodicity of Henry's painful behaviors. Did the response to Lithium mean Henry was bipolar? Probably, but not certainly. You don't have to be bipolar to get a feeling of relaxation with Lithium. But when the doctor hears the phrase, "everything is better now," it usually means that the doctor is treating the very core of the disease.

I was happy with what I had achieved. I had stumbled upon a drug which seemed to be helping Henry, and I suspected that he was bipolar, although I found no historical features to support that diagnosis. They were there, in spades, but I was not clever enough to discern them. The psychiatrist did. Maybe Henry was more open with her. His Lithium therapy had, after all, made him a much more engaging person. She recorded, as had I, a history of a self-inflicted gunshot wound in his abdomen many years ago. He told me it was an accident, and I accepted his lie. The psychiatrist obtained a history of periodic attacks of rapid speech, hyperactivity, and financial disinhibition. Henry would sometimes go on spending sprees, exhausting his financial resources. Uncontrolled spending is an important feature of bipolar disease, a manic, irresponsible behavior.

The psychiatrist continued the Lithium and added Depakote, another mood stabilizer, and Henry has done well. He remains even-tempered, free of depression, free of spending binges, and free of attacks of back pain. Henry suffered bipolar disease. There were intervals of depression, on occasion to the point of a suicide attempt. On other occasions, there were intervals of hyperactivity and disinhibition. And on others, remarkably, attacks of pain.

Why does bipolar disease express itself as painfulness? The best answer to that question is another one. Why not? Pain is a cerebral and behavioral experience just as are depression and mania. They frequently coexist in the same mind-soul. There is, without question, a high concordance of bipolar disease and painfulness. Unfortunately, this association is not widely recognized.

Ed was referred for treatment of his fibromyalgia. It came on after coronary bypass surgery. He had a rough go with the operation, developing respiratory failure sufficient to put him on a ventilator for a couple of days. He recovered and left the hospital chest-painful, as they all are, after a sternum splitting operation. His heart was restored, but his pain continued, extending to the muscles of his upper back and neck. He also suffered daily headaches. He was chronically upper body painful. He had failed to recover.

I reviewed the events of his life and concluded that the antecedent of his painfulness was cerebral injury incurred during an interval of hypoxia due to his pulmonary complications. He was on several drugs, muscle relaxants and analgesics, when I got him. I added more, a benzodiazepine and tricyclic, and he slowly got better, but he did not get well. I followed him for several months observing an incomplete response to my therapy. I elected to employ Lithium. I had not the least suspicion of bipolarity. There was no historic evidence to suggest that diagnosis, but Ed was chronically depressed and painful, and Lithium as augmentation therapy to tricyclics was warranted. On his next visit, Ed reported that his pain had diminished. "Everything is better," he said. He did very well for a few months, then an unfortunate circumstance. He suffered an unexpected financial reverse. A clue perhaps?

Unable to afford medical insurance, Ed went to the Veterans Administration hospital, where his treatment could be continued at no cost to him. The physicians there were startled at his polypharmacy. Other physicians are often dismayed by the number of drugs I employ in the treatment of the painful. I am sure other pain doctors are subject to the same sort of suspicion. Again, the mind-body dichotomy. Drugs in great number and variety are employed in the treatment of diseases such as rheumatoid arthritis, diabetes, and heart failure. These are all serious illnesses, worthy of aggressive treatment. The use of multiple drugs in unaccountable illness is, however, suspect. The VA physicians were unable to leave well enough alone. In their shoes, I suppose I might have done the same thing. They admitted Ed for drug adjustments. Removing him from my drugs, they placed him on others, equal in number but, it turned out, without effect. Ed's pain reappeared, as did his sleeplessness and depression.

He came back to me, this time in the company of his wife, begging for assistance. I slowly removed him from his Trazodone, Remeron, Ambien, and Prozac. These are good drugs for depression and insomnia, but they are rather ineffective in the treatment of pain. I resumed his prior therapy and achieved some success. It was incomplete, however. Ed didn't reach nearly the level of analgesia or well-being he had the first time. This is often the case when effective drugs are suddenly withdrawn. They don't work as well the second time as they did the first. Something has been lost.

During the course of the interviews, I got to know Ed's wife. She was a pleasant and very observant person. As I talked with her I got to know a little bit more about Ed. He was somewhat erratic and moody she said, but they had a good life, and she was happy with her husband except for one issue. They never had any money. Ed made a fine living, but periodically he would go out on spending sprees. I prevailed on Ed to see a psychiatrist. Bipolar disease, declared my consultant. He added Depakote.

Ed did handsomely for a couple of years. His psychiatrist managed his drug therapy and there was no need for my services until his pain recurred, this time in his hip. It was quite severe, and he requested my intervention. There was clear nociceptive pathology. Ed's hip joint was destroyed by arthritis. I referred him to an orthopedist. Hip replacement was done, and Ed settled in at a rehab center for a couple of weeks of physical therapy.

Sometimes when patients change doctors or enter the hospital, prior drug therapy is inadvertently discontinued. Ed, preoccupied with efforts at rehabilitation, did not realize that his Lithium and Depakote had been discarded. Nonetheless, his progress was quite satisfactory. Astonishingly, he had little pain as he progressively ambulated on his artificial hip. He left the rehabilitation center enthusiastic about his progress. He dropped by my office to thank me for referring him to the orthopedist. A wonderful doctor, Ed told me. His recovery had been almost miraculous. He had never felt so well! When it is too good to be true, it usually is. Ed, deprived of Lithium and Depakote, was entering a manic interval. I encouraged him to get back to the psychiatrist posthaste.

Grace suffered chronic low back pain. She had gone through several lumbar disc surgeries but remained painful. She had a history of recurrent depression and had even required shock therapy along the way. I viewed her depression as a certain antecedent of her painfulness. I began my treatments first with Nortriptyline and Klonopin and later Triavil, for she had a history of exposure to that drug during her many psychiatric encounters in the past. She got better, but she didn't get well. Months into her treatment I added Lithium as augmentation, hoping to get a boost to her tricyclic therapy. "Things are better," she said, and her husband acknowledged that she was indeed more even on this drug. It went nicely for quite a while and then, Lithium therapy notwithstanding, Grace's underlying bipolar disease expressed itself with an attack of mania. As typically occurs with that state of being, she experienced an incredible sense of wellness. She became supremely happy, confident, and painless. During this interval of comfort, Grace discontinued her drugs. This is rather typical behavior. Bipolar patients often discard their therapy during mania. After all, why bother? They feel so good they don't need any medicine. After a few weeks, her cycle complete, Grace's depression reappeared. Uninhibited by pharmacy, it was deep. When she chose to resume her medicine, she did it in an act of suicidal impulsivity. She took them all at once. She survived and remains now on a strange assembly of pharmaceuticals including Lithium, Nortriptyline, Klonopin, and Triavil. Polypharmacy—needful and appropriate polypharmacy.

Bipolarity, like most psychiatric illnesses, escapes precise definition. The characteristic cyclicity of mood and behavior need not occur. Psychiatrists often employ Lithium or other mood stabilizers empirically in their treatment of refractory depression. In not a few cases it is very effective, suggesting that unremitting depression, even without intervals of mania, may represent a form of bipolar disease.

The depression of bipolar disease often responds favorably not only to mood stabilizers but to conventional antidepressants such as tricyclics and SSRIs. There are exceptions, however. Sometimes the administration of an antidepressant to a bipolar patient will actually shift neural routings into an alternate behavior and induce mania. A young woman came to me for evaluation and treatment of her fibromyalgia. As is often the case with that disease, she had a history of depression in the past. It had never required treatment. It always went away on its own. I was confident that she would respond to tricyclics. I expected her treatment to be fairly simple and successful. I prescribed Nortriptyline. A few days later I received a call from her husband. She had taken his credit cards as well as her own and gone out spending, putting him in debt by several thousand dollars. Believe it or not, her pain, quite as much as her occasional depressions, was an expression of her bipolar state. She would, I was sure, respond to the addition of a mood stabilizer, and I so advised her husband. Unfortunately, I never had an opportunity to exercise my skills. He wouldn't let her come back to me.

Depression and mania. Reverse sides of the same coin. Just as we occasionally precipitate mania by the administration of tricyclic drugs to the bipolar, so do we, I suspect, sometimes precipitate depression. Not infrequently painful patients will exhibit in response to tricyclic drugs a profound, overwhelming, weeping despondency. It is a frightful thing to see, an effect perhaps not different from Prozac-generated suicide attempts. Could that behavior represent a symptom of an underlying bipolar disorder?

Arnold is one of my favorite patients. He drops by occasionally, and I always enjoy his visits, for he is a charming person. Good health has been his lot. He has a flamboyant personality, is quick-witted and energetic, and capable of working many hours a day without fatigue. He never, at least to my eye, seemed to get down. Life's reverses just didn't bother him. For a long time I thought his amazing resiliency represented some sort of capacity for denial, but I finally realized that was not the case at all.

Arnold makes lots of money and spends it all. His automobiles are expensive, convertible, and red and yellow. His clothes are as bright. He is a peacock, whether at cocktail parties, weddings, or funerals—I think it was the funeral attire that made me realize he was really on the edge. On the edge or not, he is delightful company.

Arnold rarely takes anything seriously. Only once in our encounters has there been any real intimacy. He mentioned his occasional intervals of sudden despondency. They always went away, sometimes in a few hours, sometimes in a few days. They were tolerable, but he wondered why he should be afflicted with such despair when he felt so good most of the time. And then he dismissed the question out of hand, resuming his bonhomie and jocularity, and he said no more of the matter.

Arnold has Bipolar II disorder. The range of the swings is less than in Bipolar I. In that disease depression may reach psychotic or suicidal depths, and mania the height of irresponsibility and freedom from constraint. The amplitude of swings is less in Bipolar II. They are less visible, less disturbing, and sometimes not there at all. Some bipolar patients possess, throughout their lives, a sleep-needless energized capacity for work. They are often very successful people. Arnold really didn't ask me for advice about his occasional depressions. He didn't want to pursue the issue, nor did I. He was successful and content, happy most of the time. He had a stable marriage of many years' duration. It would have been a mistake, I thought, to treat him. A life of baseline hypomania (not quite mania) is not a bad life. Leave it alone.

Not infrequently painful patients will exhibit in response to tricyclic drugs a profound, overwhelming, weeping despondency. It is a frightful thing to see.

Bipolarity II falls within the spectrum of psychiatric illness, but many times it falls also within the range of normal human behavior. Many bipolars are free of the periodic interludes of depression which may, but need not, accompany their disease. They are endowed with vigor and quite often by creativity and quick-wittedness. They can be very charming people. Their occasional disinhibited behaviors aside, they often hold positions of great responsibility. Bipolars become physicians, executives, community leaders, fighter pilots, and presidents.

They also become painful. The history of sleep-needless, hyperenergized behavior as an antecedent to painfulness is remarkable in its frequency. Many painful patients were, prior to the onset of their disease, very successful people, capable of efficiency, dispatch, and doing two or three things at once. This is quite evident in the history taking if we but search for it.

Mabel was referred to me for an evaluation of possible multiple sclerosis. She was a social worker, a church organist, and in her spare time, a designer of jewelry. Her hysterectomy had been done about five years before. Six weeks to the day after that event, she suffered for the first time a siege of headaches. An MRI of the brain was done because cerebral aneurysm was suspect. None was found, but the imaging study showed a few patchy subcortical white spots. These lesions are sometimes indicative of multiple sclerosis, but more often they mean nothing (or at least nothing we yet understand). In many cases they are an irrelevant and innocuous finding. Nonetheless, the specter of multiple sclerosis had been raised. As time went by, she developed some symptoms of that disease. She acquired an intermittent hand tremor, worse with intention, as in writing. Over the course of several years' observation, her MRIs did not change, and her clinical behaviors but little. She developed restless legs and periodically experienced sensations of fatigue. On those occasions she would notice that her gait was impaired. Her legs felt weak, and she had trouble going up stairs. These attacks came in waves, periodically, every couple of months, and during them her tremor would worsen. She exhibited another form of periodicity. Once a month, during ovulation, she would experience a recurrence of headaches, by now recognized as a very typical migraine. Headache is hardly a symptom of multiple sclerosis, but weakness, fatigue, and tremor are. She also had another symptom that suggested multiple sclerosis. She was heat-sensitive. A hot bath would produce profound fatigue and sometimes she would even lose bladder control and urinate on herself.

I first saw her during an interval of wellness, and her neurologic exam, aside from a very fine, almost indiscernible tremor in her hands was quite normal. Her gait was unencumbered, her muscle strength good. There was no visual disturbance, and her cognition was beyond normal. Sharp as a tack and creative, she wrote poetry, she said, and had some pieces published.

Multiple sclerosis it could be, but there was no way to be sure of that. The disease may be relentlessly progressive, but more often it is characterized by random attacks of neurologic dysfunction.

These attacks are quite erratic in their appearance, recurring over many years. Multiple sclerosis is a recurrent disease, but it is not a cyclical disease. There is a difference. My young patient was cycling. Her migraines occurred once a month like clockwork. More irregularly, every couple of months or so, she would suffer restless legs, worsening tremor, and fatigue. During these interludes she also experienced pain—in the back with a burning sensation down her legs. She also experienced hypersomnolence, sleeping twelve or fourteen hours a day. During wellness she needed little sleep: a few hours would do just fine. I asked about her mood, whether it cycled also. She said she was unaware of it, but acknowledged that her husband could identify a spell at its onset by a change in her disposition. He treated her with kid gloves during these intervals, she said, but no, she never experienced any real sense of despondency.

Alternate behaviors, cycling periodic behaviors. Migraine once a month and at longer, less predictable intervals, fatigue, tremor, restless legs, change in temperament, and pain. Her disease might have been a form of the premenstrual syndrome. Uterus-deprived but with an intact pituitary and ovarian axis, she was subject to hormonal shifts and their effect on behavior. I suspect, however, that my beautiful, bright, creative and energized young patient had Bipolar II disease. Why it should first appear six weeks after a hysterectomy is unknown, but it certainly is not coincidence. Intercurrent illness and surgeries often expose latent diseases into display, be these migraine, bipolarity, or multiple sclerosis.

Mabel's life was, most of the time, one of contentment and great effectiveness. The physician must take care when treating such patients. I did elect to try, in turn, a couple of drugs. Depakote and Topamax are both mood stabilizers and also effective in the prevention of migraine. Neither worked. Her cyclic headaches, fatigue, and pain continued. I finally gave Mabel my best judgment—wait it out.

Where does multiple sclerosis fit in the equation? Possibly, maybe even probably there, taking its time to show its face. Her disease or diseases will, I am sure, sooner or later declare themselves. In which form or mixture I can only guess. She may evolve into a manic interval, or a major depression, or a true giveaway sign of multiple sclerosis such as double vision, paralysis, or sensory loss. She may even manifest conversion disorder as a symptom of that disease. Fragments, partials, *formes fruste*, and comorbidities. There is a continuum. Behavior and biology are inseparable.

Clyde was forty when I first saw him. He was quite an intelligent man. His quick-thinking, quick-acting behaviors were evident from the very beginning. In our conversation, he never paused for reflection. His responses were instantaneous, and there was great richness and variety in his thought. He acknowledged that he had an active mind and suggested that he probably inherited it from his mother, who was bipolar. He denied any history of depression. To the contrary, he told me, he was always wired and upbeat, and in his job of selling insurance, that was quite an asset.

About five years before we met, he began to experience pain in his left ear. At first it was intermittent, but it gradually became incessant, and Clyde consulted several otologists. None could find any abnormality of the ear. A couple of them did suggest that he might be experiencing pain referred from his temporomandibular joint. They advised consultation with an oral surgeon. An operation was performed, but it did not relieve the pain. It continued and spread to his posterior skull, neck, and left face. It became associatied, remarkably, with a most unusual tinnitus, a sound emanating within the ear.

Tinnitus is a common disorder. It is often identified as the sound of crickets chirping. Not so in Clyde. His was a knocking sound, occurring pulse-like but not synchronous with his heartbeat. It occurred with lesser frequency, about twenty times a minute, like a slow clock ticking in his head. In most patients with tinnitus there is some discernible loss of auditory acuity. Clyde's hearing, however, was quite good.

Was Clyde's tinnitus an auditory hallucination, a creation of his overactive mind? Or a form of obsession, a thought and sensation that simply would not go away? Or a delusion, a twisted and malformed thought perhaps? If not one of these, I suspected at least something like them.

Clyde had more surgery. Polyps were removed from his sinuses, but without benefit. Then a repair of his nasal septum, deviated perhaps by some remote trauma. That didn't work either. Clyde decided to give up on doctors and live with his discomfort and the strange sound emanating within his ear.

He got by well enough. He was still energetic, little needful of sleep, and economically and socially comfortable. Still, he confided to me, he always knew that something was wrong. Not just in his ear, but in his mind. He felt subject to thought racing and his brain was so full of ideas that he frequently felt overwhelmed. He also recognized his impulsivity, his propensity to go out and buy things he didn't need.

Several years into his illness, Clyde experienced a pain far removed from his ear. It was in his back and radiated into his leg. He consulted an orthopedist, and an MRI identified a ruptured disc compressing the fifth lumbar nerve. The surgeon opted for conservative care, suggesting an interval of bedrest before pursuing any kind of intervention. Within a couple of weeks, Clyde's back pain abated, but as it did, his ear pain worsened.

I have written before of the curious capacity of new pains to resurrect old ones. Just why and how this should happen, and it happens a lot, I will leave to the reader's imagination.

I have written before of the curious capacity of new pains to resurrect old ones. Just why and how this should happen, and it happens a lot, I will leave to the reader's imagination. I will only point out the paradox. Clyde's back, with a ruptured disc impinging on a nerve, should have continued to hurt but didn't. At the same time, his ear, which was normal, and shouldn't have hurt at all, became even more painful.

I delighted in his company. His intelligence and wit were extraordinary. After our first interview he suggested to me, "Hey, you are quick. You are just like me. I think I trust you." No ingratiation this, just two hypomanic souls finding comfort with each other. We got on in a big way. I knew I would not find pathologic anatomy to account for Clyde's syndrome of painfulness and tinnitis. Physicians more expert than I in diseases of the ear and face had had no luck at all. Scant chance that I would succeed where they failed. Clyde's pain and tinnitis were not coming from his organ of audition. They were coming from his mind.

I prescribed Imipramine and Klonopin. In a short while Clyde began to sleep more and better. He reported that when he awoke in the morning, there was a certain sense of equilibrium and comfort that he had not known before. He offered a statement of succinctness and great meaning. "Now, I can think better." Remarkable how often I hear this phrase when the painful patient starts getting better. The experience of pain is, without question, related to the experience of thought.

I added Lithium. I simply had to. I couldn't resist.

"Everything is better now," he said, "ever better."

"The sound in your ear. Is it still there?"

"Yes, it's there, and the pain is still there, but they just don't seem to bother me as much."

"Are my drugs slowing you down? Do you feel sedated?"

"Nope, I am still going fast."

Perfect is the enemy of the good. Clyde's response wasn't perfect. It was merely very good. He and I elected to catch our breath and continue his medicines without, at least for a while, any more experimentations. It went nicely for several weeks, but then Clyde started losing ground. His pain became a little worse, his tinnitis more distracting, and his sleep less restorative.

Ritalin certainly wasn't nonsensical therapy, but it was, I admit, a stretch. There was just something about Clyde's thought-racing and his inability to really organize his ideas that suggested the possibility of attention deficit disorder. It does occur in the adult, and it is remarkable how well Ritalin can work. It was worth a shot. Clyde got two things out of Ritalin, both bad. He lost his appetite, and he didn't need to do that. He was plenty skinny enough. He also experienced, for the first time in his life, migraine headaches. He suffered attacks of unilateral pain associated with nausea and blurred vision. Ritalin has an effect similar to amphetamine, a stimulant and vasoactive substance that is sometimes a migraine trigger. Interestingly, Clyde's headaches occurred exclusively on his left, ear-painful side, never on his right. A coincidence perhaps, or did it represent the incorporation and recruitment of a prior painful experience into the expression of migraine?

Ritalin didn't work, but it was worth a try. Pain does occur with neuropsychiatric comorbidities even though we have to accept that these may exist in fragmentary form. ADD it could have been, but it wasn't. It was time to move on to other drugs. But which? Perhaps an antipsychotic, a thought-altering drug. I believed that Clyde's pain and tinnitis represented a thought warp, but caution was in order. Most of Clyde's thoughts were good. Very good indeed. I didn't want to meddle with something working that well. Better to try another avenue, perhaps another mood stabilizer on top of Lithium. There were many choices, Tegretol, Neurontin, Depakote, or Topamax. I suspected one would work, but I didn't know which. I tried Topamax. The drug has a common side effect. It produces numbness and tingling, almost always in the extremities. Clyde, as I should have expected, experienced a different sort of reaction. He did become numb, but only in his nose. His richly innervated and close-to-the-brain nose tingled, predominantly, of course, on the left side.

One of the problems in the treatment of pain, as if we didn't have enough already, is the abundance of potentially helpful drugs.

Clyde, with his capacity for upbeat and volatile thought, suggested, "Maybe it's working. Maybe it will move around and make my ear numb."

"No, Clyde, I don't think it will work that way." Deep down, though, I wondered. Almost anything can happen in the painful patient. Naaahh. No way.

One of the problems in the treatment of pain, as if we didn't have enough already, is the abundance of potentially helpful drugs. There are some two hundred major neuropsychiatric drugs in current usage, and most of them are effective for pain. A surfeit of riches. A group of new drugs, the atypical antipsychotics, hold great promise. They were greeted with enthusiasm because they offered a treatment choice for schizophrenia without the risk of tremors and rigidity. We now recognize, several years into their existence, that they are much more than that. They are a latter day Triavil, useful for many diseases—psychosis, depression, and bipolar disease.

I gave him Zyprexa. Starting low and slow, I prescribed only 2.5 milligrams daily. Nothing happened at first, but as the dosage increased, Clyde got well. It didn't take long, a month or so. His pain and tinnitus progressively diminished. They didn't go completely away, however. Painfulness and its attendants only rarely go away totally in response to drug therapy, but they can be vastly and comfortably diminished. They were in Clyde.

Neuropsychiatric illnesses, in their interminglings and the diversity of their effects, exhibit an incredible variety of display. There is, nonetheless, a certain constancy when the right drug kicks in. Some depressives, not a few at all, who respond to therapy (particularly Prozac) employ a very singular phrase in their descriptions—"I am even now." Painful patients, when they respond to drug therapy, remark with astonishing frequency, "I can think better now."

"Everything is better." "I am even now." "I can think better now." Profound in meaning, these words tell us that we are down there with the neurotransmitters, influencing, in a manner quite beyond our comprehension, the mind-soul and its endeavors.

Louise suffered attacks of pain in the right ankle. They would last for a few days, and they occurred randomly, something on the order of three or four times a year. Her rheumatologist saw her several times, once during an attack of pain. He discerned signs of inflammation, with heat, redness, and pain in the ankle. He could not, however, find any evidence of rheumatologic disorder in his laboratory testing. Anti-inflammatory drugs were ineffective and so was cortisone. Taken with the patient's unusual behaviors and curious that they might relate in some manner to her pain, he referred her to me.

Thin and graceful, she was well-groomed and quick, lightning quick. She was a soccer mom, she said. Three kids and a Dodge van. She was a court reporter and very good at it. The best in northern Alabama, she told me. She had a waiting list for depositions. She was lean, and she reveled in it. She jogged three miles each day and did three hundred sit-ups (half in the morning, half in the evening). She read her Bible for an hour each day, maintained successful employment, and cared for her husband, children, and home without any kind of domestic assistance. "How in the world do you get that all in?" It was easy, she told me. She just never required much sleep. Three hours was plenty. The remainder of the day was sufficient for her tasks.

She was one of the most restless creatures I have ever seen. Simply watching her sit was an uncomfortable experience. She constantly crossed one leg over the other, back and forth, all the while tapping her fingers on her knee. At rest she was a metabolic blast furnace, and even that state of relative repose could not be sustained for any length of time. She often interrupted conversation by standing and pacing back and forth as I attempted to talk with her. She was razor sharp and quick as a hiccup. She answered my questions before I could finish asking them. I couldn't keep up with her, and I am not slow. Her motoric skills were as super-charged as her verbal ones. She chewed her gum with ear-numbing rapidity. She seemed, when I could hold her down for a bit, to be even-tempered. She denied any moodiness or depression. There was no evidence of disordered thought. The only blot on her exceptional, speeded life was the occasional occurrence of inexplicable ankle pain.

I prescribed Neurontin and advised her that the attacks were so infrequent that it might be months before we knew whether the drug was working. She was not enthusiastic. She lived some distance away, and visits to my office were inconvenient. She would like to pursue the treatment, she said, as she winked at me, but she really was awfully busy. We terminated our relationship.

How will it all end up? I don't really know, but I have some suspicion. Her pain is recurrent and kindling. Somewhere along the way it will lose its periodicity and manifest as relentless painfulness. When this happens her life will, I believe, begin to unravel. She may evolve into some form of bipolar disease with manic and disinhibited behavior or, perhaps more likely, she will become depressed (depression is common, mania is not). When that happens she will, for the first time in her life, experience fatigue. She will become fat and disinterested in jogging and sit-ups and her job. Her subcortical brain's internal gyroscope, angled so strongly toward sleepless hyperactivity, will, sooner or later, tilt equally dramatically in the opposite direction. When that happens, all the good things—her leanness, her energy, and her quickness—will transmogrify into lethargic apathy, despondency, and chronic pain. Then, and perhaps only then, will she respond to drug therapy. It is difficult to treat wellness, and Louise, save for occasional ankle pain, was supremely well. Her neuronal activity was efficient and gainful and not to be bothered with any kind of pharmacologic intervention. When the wheels come off, however, and her neuronal routing is confused and inefficient, it will accept the appropriate chemical or combination of chemicals to nudge it back where it belongs.

CHAPTER FIFTEEN

Chronic Fatigue

D arlene was new to the city. She was a stockbroker and an attractive, poised, and forceful young woman. She began our conversation by asking me, "Do you know anything about dysautonomia?"

"A little maybe. I am not sure anybody knows much about it."

"I have chronic fatigue and dysautonomia. The doctors in St. Louis finally got it worked out. They want to keep an eye on me, and I will go back there a couple of times a year, but I need a primary care physician."

"Tell me about it."

"About two years ago I developed fibromyalgia. I had constant dull pain in my neck and shoulders. I was tired all the time, and I couldn't sleep at night. My doctor gave me sleeping pills and told me to exercise."

"Did that help?"

"No, I was too tired to exercise. Whenever I did, I would feel faint. I would suddenly break out in a sweat, and when that happened, I felt like I was losing it, like I was passing out. Sometimes I would be so weak I could hardly walk. The doctor did some blood tests and told me I had mononucleosis and the chronic fatigue syndrome."

"What did he do then?"

"He told me to rest, and the symptoms would probably go away."

"Did they?"

"No, they just got worse. I kept feeling like I was blacking out. It was so bad one time that I went to the emergency room. The doctors there told me that my pulse was thirty, and my blood pressure ninety over sixty. They called in a cardiologist, and after he checked me over, he told me I had dysautonomia. He put in a heart pacemaker."

Dysautonomia, as the name suggests, is a disorder of the neural system that regulates cardiac and visceral activity. It is, in a sense, a functional disease. A heart which is anatomically normal behaves in a dysfunctional manner just as the bowels behave dysfunctionally in the patient with the irritable bowel syndrome. That disease is one of discomfort and inconvenience. Cardiac dysautonomia, however, is a much more threatening illness. A pulse rate of thirty is always taken seriously. A heart rate that slow can certainly cause faintness and fatigue. The insertion of a cardiac pacemaker was warranted. The procedure has been done countless times, usually in the elderly who suffer heart disease. Not many thirty-two-year-olds require pacemakers, though.

"I am sure you felt better with a pacemaker."

"Not really. My heart rate stayed up, but I didn't get any better. I kept feeling like I was fainting. My fatigue was just terrible. I couldn't think right, and I had a bad problem with my memory. I was in a brain fog all the time. It was really hard to work."

Dysautonomia, and with it, chronic fatigue. Appropriately diagnosed and appropriately treated but without success. The heart rhythm was restored, but the patient did not improve—a failure to recover syndrome if there ever was one. I asked Darlene to continue.

"I decided to go to another cardiologist."

"That sounds like a good idea."

"He was an expert in dysautonomia. He put me on a tilt table and measured my pulse and blood pressure in different positions and after exercise. I wore a heart monitor for twenty-four hours, and when it was all done, he gave me a drug called Norpace."

"Did that work? Did you feel better?"

"Yes, I did, but it took a long time. It was a couple of months before I started getting well, but I did finally. My energy came back, and my fibromyalgia improved. I felt well enough to start working again. I left St. Louis and relocated here to start over."

"So maybe you didn't really need the pacemaker after all."

"That's what the doctor said. He took it out."

Wow! A thirty-two-year-old woman subjected to a pacemaker in, then a pacemaker out—and then exquisite control of her complex symptoms with a cardiac drug, little-used now. I searched for information about Norpace and the treatment of fatigue, but I couldn't find any. No matter, the drug seemed to be working. Leave well enough alone. I told Darlene I would be happy to see her if problems arose. She could return to St. Louis periodically for follow-up.

I kept my real thoughts to myself. Was her disease in the heart or was it in the mind? A pacemaker restored the heart rhythm but didn't help the patient. Her slow heart rate and low blood pressure were, I suspected, not the cause of her illness. They were symptoms of it. Her response to Norpace was queer. It is a quick-acting drug. Within hours, days at most, its effect should be evident. In Darlene it took months to start working. I pushed a little harder.

"Do you have a problem with depression?"

"Yes, I'm on Prozac."

"Is it working?"

"Yes, very well. I need the Prozac. If I stop it for a few days, the depression comes back. When I take it, I do okay, but I still have trouble sleeping. Every time I get in bed at night, my legs start jerking. They told me it is called restless legs."

"How long have you had trouble sleeping?"

"As far back as I can remember. Everybody in my family has trouble sleeping. They all have restless legs."

"Do any of them have trouble with pain, fatigue, or depression?"

"No, they are all healthy. We are just a family of poor sleepers."

"I suppose you have taken many kinds of sleeping pills?"

"Yes, I have tried several of them, but none really worked. When I first got sick and was so fatigued and sleepy all the time, they did a sleep study and told me I had sleep apnea. It was a severe case, and the doctors advised an operation to open up the back of my throat so I could breathe better at night."

"Did it work?"

"Yes, at first I slept well, but when I developed dysautonomia a few months later, the insomnia came back."

Sleep apnea occurs in persons, usually males, with obesity and with thick, heavy necks. Darlene had the neck of a swan. Her disordered sleep notwithstanding, Darlene was almost well when I first saw her. Prozac and Norpace had cured her. A cardinal rule, in dealing with the human machine, is to leave it alone when it is working well. I told Darlene I would not suggest any change in her medicines, but I had a few more questions if she was willing to talk about her personal life.

"Yes, ask me anything you want."

"Are you married? Do you have children?"

"No to both. I got married when I was twenty-five and divorced when I was twenty-eight. I enjoyed my career more than my marriage."

"When did your depression first appear?"

"About the time I developed fibromyalgia and fatigue."

"What was going on in your life at that time? Were you happy in your work, in your relationships?"

"Yes, I was very happy. I was doing well and making a good living, but I did have a problem with my boss. He had a thing for me, and he was pretty aggressive. He touched me a lot. It got very frustrating. I wish I had said something about it earlier."

"What do you mean?"

"One day, after work when everyone was gone, he tried to have sex with me. I fought him off, but it was pretty frightening."

"When did this occur?"

"Right before I got sick."

An assault on that most personal and private of our behaviors can be an event of catastrophic consequence. It is, however, perhaps too easy and too convenient to ascribe diseases such as chronic pain and chronic fatigue to unfortunate sexual encounters. We have to keep it in perspective. Is it reasonable to relate the remarkable development of her illness to a single unsuccessful sexual assault? As is often the case in patients with chronic pain (and chronic fatigue), there is more going on than meets the eye. It wasn't just the assault that made Darlene ill. It was the harassment complaint that followed. It became public in short order. Lines were drawn, and Darlene found some new friends, but she lost a lot of old ones. Management circled the wagons, and Darlene became a pariah. The violated became the violator. In the end, after several months of negotiations and confrontations, her boss was reprimanded. Darlene was given a financial settlement and advised to relocate to another city.

I thanked Darlene for sharing her story with me. She was to continue her Prozac and Norpace. I advised her to check back periodically. I had a suspicion, which I did not share with her, that her recovery represented more of a spontaneous remission than a pharmacologic effect.

She returned a couple of months later. Her career was going nicely, but her sleeplessness was becoming more of a problem. I inquired if she had ever taken the drug Klonopin. She had not. It worked pretty well at first (most of the drugs work pretty well at first, sustaining their benefit is another matter). She began to experience sedation from the drug, and her depression worsened. I told her to discard the Klonopin and to increase the Prozac dosage. A few weeks later she awoke feeling very unwell and nauseated. She dressed and went out to her car and then collapsed. A neighbor found her and brought her to my office. She was drenched with sweat, unsteady on her feet, and disoriented. Her blood pressure was eighty over fifty, and her pulse forty beats per minute.

Her electrocardiogram, aside from the slow rate, was normal. She rested for a while and then took a softdrink and gradually improved, even though her blood pressure and pulse had changed not at all. When she came fully to her senses, I offered her hospital admission and consultation with a cardiologist, an electrophysiologist skillful in the treatment of dysautonomia. Perhaps he could solve the riddle that others had so clearly failed to do. Maybe Darlene recognized that this offering was less than enthusiastic. I didn't think we were going to solve her mind disease by attacking its target organ, the heart.

"No, no more heart stuff. I would like to just go home and rest."

"That's okay with me, Darlene. You are sick, but you are not dying. You have been like this many times before, and you have recovered. You can go home, but keep in touch with me and let's meet again next week to go over this thing again."

I looked forward to her next visit, perhaps selfishly. For the first time in my encounters with this woman, I did not have to be obedient to that which had gone before. The drugs were not working. I was going to get my chance.

Pain and fatigue carry the same antecedents. Both are the product of life experiences which so alter the integrity of the mind that they invite maladaptive and inefficient clinical behavior.

She looked better when I saw her, but not a lot. Her fatigue had returned full force, and her movements were cautious. Standing up rapidly made her feel faint. Her blood pressure and her pulse were still low. I told her to discard the Norpace. She had already done it, she told me.

"It wasn't working. I don't think it ever worked."

Which drug to use? Many have been employed in the treatment of fatigue. The SSRIs can be helpful, but she was already on one of those. Ritalin can be used, but it is a controlled substance, and some authorities look askance at its use in the treatment of fatigue, a second class disorder in the minds of many. The tricyclics are frequently employed, but one of their major side effects is fatigue. Nonetheless, she had never taken one before, so I gave her Nortriptyline. If it did nothing but help her sleep, that would be useful. It didn't work at all. Darlene felt worse after she took it.

I chose Topamax. It is a new drug, and its clinical indications are still uncertain, but it is potentially useful in a variety of disorders. It can relieve essential tremor. It is an antimanic drug and perhaps antidepressant. It is an impulse-controlling agent. Explosive behavior can sometimes be managed with Topamax. It is often used in the treatment of chronic pain of all origins, and it can be very effective in preventing migraine. I had no certain knowledge that Topamax could be helpful in the treatment of chronic fatigue, but I knew that Darlene was off the diagnostic tables—way off. She was afflicted with a very complex illness, and it was destructive to the simplest acts of her existence. Just think about it—lifelong insomnia, restless legs, sleep apnea, chronic fatigue, fibromyalgia, dysautonomia, depression, and migraine (she had that disease also) were all comorbid in a single young woman!

Within a week, Darlene was restored. Her fatigue, her pain, her faints, her insomnia, and her restless legs were gone. It was a clinical miracle—they do happen. There is a drug out there, as I have said before, for almost everybody. Darlene remains well four years later. Prozac and Topamax (a strange form of polypharmacy if there ever was one) cured her. Will it be sustained? I have no idea.

The chronic fatigue syndrome (CFS) and the chronic pain syndrome are one and the same illness. Most patients with CFS suffer painfulness, most commonly in the form of fibromyalgia or headaches, and patients with chronic pain are almost invariably fatigued. For a while, we believed that CFS was an infectious disease. Many patients with the disorder had evidence of prior infection with the mononucleosis virus. That was a hopeful discovery because it offered the possibility that a mind-soul disease could actually be caused by a virus. It offered an easy answer to a complex problem, but it was not to be. Most (not all) physicians have long discarded the notion that chronic fatigue is due to mononucleosis. Rest in peace, mononucleosis theory. It is highly unlikely that such a complex behavioral disorder as chronic fatigue could be due to a single type of virus. No one has seriously suggested, thank heavens, that diseases such as depression and chronic pain are infectious in origin. All the evidence points to something else.

Pain and fatigue carry the same antecedents. Both are the product of life experiences which so alter the integrity of the mind that they invite maladaptive and inefficient clinical behavior. They share the same symptoms (identifiers). Both are attended by sleeplessness, depression, and cognitive impairment. Chronic pain is responsive to a great number of pharmaceuticals. Chronic fatigue, however, is a much more difficult disease to treat. There are fewer drugs for the treatment of fatigue than there are for chronic pain. With the advent of the new pharmacy, that may be changing. Topamax was certainly effective in treating Darlene's fatigue. Will that turn out to be the breakthrough drug?

A curious feature of CFS is its frequent association with dysautonomia, but even here, the distinction between pain and fatigue is blurred. Patients with chronic pain are subject to dysautonomia. The irritable bowel syndrome, reflex sympathetic dystrophy, and migraine are all disorders of, and I will coin a word here, *regional* dysautonomia. Autonomic activity in the blood vessels of the head is disordered in migraine. It is disordered in the extremities in reflex sympathetic dystrophy. In the irritable bowel syndrome, autonomic control of the movements of the intestines is highly disturbed. Patients with chronic fatigue also suffer regional dysautonomia, but the target organ is the heart. Pulse rate, blood pressure, and cardiac output are altered, and that has dire consequence for both the mind and the body. Thus, faintness, sweats, and certainly fatigue. Does this mean that chronic fatigue is a cardiac disease? It is an attractive idea, and another hopeful one, for it invites a definitive treatment. It is rather easy to restore the heart rhythm. It is much more difficult to restore the mind. Darlene's slow pulse was corrected with a pacemaker. Her symptoms improved not at all.

Cardiac dysautonomia is common in chronic fatigue, less in chronic pain. Nonetheless, it does occur. Painful patients are often subject to lightheadedness and faints due to irregular pulse and blood pressure. Only rarely, however, are these symptoms severe enough to warrant the dramatic kind of intervention that Darlene required.

Susan suffered fatigue and, with it, dysautonomia. She became ill after an unpleasant vacation with her parents. Her office was being remodeled, and she was exposed to irritating dust and fumes. She developed a cough and respiratory inflammation, perhaps allergic, and then evolved into fatigue, insomnia, fibromyalgia, and wildly irregular heart rhythms with recurring, faint-producing tachy-cardias. I tried several drugs, some for the mind and some for the heart, but they were ineffective. I referred her to a cardiologist who advised an ablation procedure. The heart is catheterized and radiofrequency impulses are directed to the wall of the heart chamber destroying those neural pathways responsible for the irregular rhythms. She was awaiting the procedure when I called her and told her there was a new drug, Topamax, that I would like to try. She was eager and willing. I wish it had a happy ending, but it did not. She could not tolerate the Topamax. It was sedating, and she had to discard it. Nearly all the drugs work on somebody. Very few work on everybody. It is a fact of life, and we just have to accept it. Susan had her ablation procedure. Her rapid heart rhythms were arrested, but her fatigue improved not at all.

Russell experienced progressive pain in his right shoulder. His pain was due to an impingement syndrome, the constriction of the tendons of the joint. Surgery was performed to release the constriction, and he did well. Then a few months later, while jogging, he tripped and fell against his right shoulder, damaging it again and fracturing the adjacent collarbone. A redo of the operation to repair the shoulder, by now a real mess, was performed. Russell recovered more slowly from this surgery, but with time his shoulder became painless and mobile. He then developed an unrelated and seemingly trivial problem, a cyst on one of the tendons of his right hand. It was grape sized and painless, but it impaired the movement of his thumb. His orthopedist performed an operation, quite small in scope compared with the previous surgeries, and the cyst was removed. This time Russell failed to recover. The wound was slow to heal, and within a couple of weeks his hand was swollen, sweaty, livid, and painful. The orthopedist diagnosed reflex sympathetic dystrophy.

Few diagnoses are as frightful. Russell was alarmed by the prospect of a withered, useless, and painful hand. He could not understand, he told me, how he could survive major injuries to his shoulder and then be brought down by repair of a simple cyst. Nor could I, but I suspected there was an answer. There is usually an answer.

"This thing has really gotten me down. I feel exhausted. I have never been this tired before."

"Are you depressed? Do you feel sad or despondent?"

"No, I am not depressed. I'm frustrated, and I am really angry that this has happened to me. I have had a good life. Now I am not sure what I am going to do."

"Tell me about your fatigue. What is it like?"

"I'm exhausted when I wake up. It is like I have never been to sleep. It takes me a long time to clean up and get dressed in the morning. I don't sleep well. My legs have started jerking at night when I try to sleep. I don't know what in the world that means."

"How is your appetite?"

"I don't have any. I am too tired to eat."

"Your sexual energy?"

"Zip."

"But you are not depressed?"

"Nope, I don't feel sad. I just feel tired. I am too tired to even think. I don't read any more. I can't seem to remember. Lots of times I feel like I am about to faint. I've never gone all the way out, but many times I have to hold on to something to keep from falling. It will just come all over me. My face will turn red—my wife says almost blue sometimes—and I will be drenched with sweat."

"It almost sounds like your face turns the same color as your hand."

"That is exactly right! My wife says my face looks like my hand."

"How much pain do you have in your hand?"

"Ibuprofen does a pretty good job with it. The pain is not too bad, but the fatigue is horrible. I'm worthless. I don't know if I will be able to work any more, and I have a young son to educate."

"Tell me about your son."

"I married late. My wife is a school teacher, and our son is four years old."

"What did you do for a living?"

"I was in manufacturing. I started with a company out of engineering school. I stayed there for twenty-five years."

"Are you still there?"

"No, we were bought out, and I decided to leave."

"After twenty-five years?"

"Yes, I am still a young man, and I wanted to start my own business."

"Were you happy with that decision?"

"Yes, I think so. I have always wanted to be on my own."

"Was there a conflict when you left?"

"Yes, there was, I will admit. I didn't like the new manager, and he didn't like me. If it hadn't been for that, I probably would have stayed."

Chronic pain and chronic fatigue are not random occurrences. They obey a tempo imposed by life events. That which disturbs the mind disturbs also the body. Russell was in mid-life and in good health when he experienced a stressor in the form of a forced and unhappy job change. The resiliency of his infrastructure was adequate to that challenge, and for a while to the others which followed. A damaged and painful shoulder was repaired without event. And then a more serious injury. Another operation and slow recovery. The infrastructure was intact, but the experience of pain in the right upper extremity had been kindled. Then another insult, albeit a small one, the excision of a cyst in the hand. This time Russell failed to recover, and he evolved into a syndrome of chronic fatigue and chronic pain. He experienced with these, dysautonomia. His sweatiness, flushing, and faintness represented a cardiac dysautonomia. His painful, cold, and discolored hand represented regional dysautonomia in the form of reflex sympathetic dystrophy. Chronic fatigue, chronic pain, and dysautonomia, cardiac and regional, all together very likely the product of a series of unfortunate life events.

Chronic pain invites, perhaps as no other disease does, the employ of our imagination in its understanding. I will offer, without apology, a bit of speculation. Russell's cyst, which was the straw that broke the camel's back, was on his right hand, the same side as his twice-damaged and painful shoulder. The memory of those events, recently acquired, was viable and strong. Is it possible that the recurrent experience of pain in the right shoulder invited pain (reflex sympathetic dystrophy) in the hand of the same extremity? What would have happened if Russell's cyst had been on his left rather than his right hand? Would brain analgesic systems, those unkindled by previous experiences on the other side of the body, have successfully modulated the painful signal? Think about it.

CHAPTER SIXTEEN

Migraine

M igraine is a disease of periodic headaches separated by intervals of wellness. That is the briefest and possibly the best definition we have for the disease. There are, of course, more elaborate diagnostic criteria for migraine. The location, duration, and character of the pain, and the variety of accompaniments that attend the painful interval allow us, at least in typical cases, to make a diagnosis of migraine with relative ease. In clinical medicine, however, most patients are not typical, and the distinction between migraine and other forms of headache can be quite difficult. Some of the difficulty is of our own making. In our efforts to define migraine on the basis of its painful characteristics, we overlook the cardinal feature of the disease, that it goes away, and between attacks the patient is quite well.

The typical migraine attack, formerly called classic migraine, but now migraine with aura (more descriptive, but it does lack flair), begins with a prodromal or aural experience. This is usually a change in mood or temperament, often a sense of restlessness or despondency. The senses of taste and smell may be disordered during the migraine prodrome, but it is vision that is most often disturbed. The migraine aura may consist of scintillations, sparkling lights across the field of gaze. A blind spot, typically geometric and polyangular in configuration, may appear. This *scotoma*, frequently bordered by scintillations, may remain fixed in visual space, but more often it expands in size and migrates from one segment of the visual field to another, crossing left-right boundaries. Visual field defects may occur. This is the effect of a drape moving across one half of the vision producing a *hemianopia*. Sometimes only a quarter of vision is lost, a *quadrantanopia*. Curiously, the visual effects of migraine may originate either in the eye or in the brain. Ocular migraine, a loss of central vision (the scotoma), is due to disturbance in the retina, where vision to both sides is subserved. Hemianopic migraine is due to disturbance in the brain, where vision to each side is subserved by the opposite half of the occipital cortex. Regardless, the visual effects of migraine, whether originating in the retina or the cortex are, almost invariably, geometric hallucinations of vision. Always inanimate, there is never a hallucination of people, places, or recognizable things. Remarkable when you think about it. The dysfunctional brain of migraine expresses itself, at least visually, in abstract structural configurations. This occurs in no other disease. It is unique to migraine.

Somatic as well as visual sensation is disordered in the migraine aura, usually in a very lateralized manner. A sense of localized numbness and tingling is often a prodromal experience. It is usually confined to one side of the face but sometimes extends to the hand. Motor function is disturbed also, and it too is unilateral, consisting of transient weakness, usually in one arm. The function of speech, a unilateral left brain attribute, is frequently impaired.

The temporal pattern of prodromal events is erratic. Most occur before the pain, but some during it. Regardless, the visual and auditory senses remain at attention throughout the headache. Exposure to light and sound worsen pain. The migraineur is *photosonophobic*. Thus, the quiet dark room offers refuge.

When the migraine headache does occur, it can be excruciating. It is typically unilateral (but occasionally bilateral) and pulsatile. Autonomic function is disordered with nausea, vomiting, and sometimes diarrhea. Transient hypertension may occur. Blood pressure may reach astronomical levels during a migraine attack. Thought may be disordered. A confusional interval as a manifestation of migraine is well known, as is the occasional transient ablation of recent memory, the global amnesia syndrome. Not only are thought and memory disordered, so is impulse control. During an attack, migraineurs sometimes contemplate suicide and on not a few occasions, perform it successfully.

Migraine, like so many painful diseases, is intimately related to sleep. Cluster headaches occur predominantly, and often exclusively, at night. Other forms of migraine have nocturnal predilection. Sometimes the headache appears full force immediately on awakening from sleep. On the other hand, demonstrating the mind's capacity for paradox, recovery from migraine is frequently effected through the aegis of sleep. Sleep cures migraine, and that clinical observation has not received the attention it deserves. The cardinal features of the disease are, in the minds of most, the complex prodrome, the unilaterality of headache, and the occurrence of photosonophobia. Equally diagnostic, however, is the fact that it is relieved by sleep. No other painful state is so responsive to taking a nap.

The migraineur is certainly subject to change in the environment, internal or external. Emotional stress can generate a migraine attack as can hormonal changes; the phenomenon of menstrual migraine is quite common. A change in the weather with lower barometric pressure may induce migraine. Interestingly, many other forms of pain are climatic sensitive. Arthritis and fibromyalgia are certainly examples. Some foods, especially those prepared by fermentation (such as wine and cheese), may cause headache. Nearby pains, as I have said, may provoke migraine. A neck sprain or an abscessed tooth not infrequently precipitate an attack.

Migraine is not invariably associated with severe headache. Sometimes the pain can be modest in severity and sometimes not there at all. The strange accompaniments can be predominant and occasionally the only expression of the disease. Ophthalmic migraine is associated with evanescent scotoma unaccompanied by headaches. Transient numbness and weakness in an extremity, events which mimic an impending stroke, can be due to migraine and may occur in the absence of any headache at all. Partials, fragments, *formes fruste*, if you will.

There are a number of drugs available for the treatment of migraine. Ergot, a vasoconstrictor (and also a dopamine stimulating drug), has long been used to abort head pain. Other drugs known collectively as triptans are also vasoconstrictors (and serotonin stimulating drugs). The first of these was Imitrex, followed by

Zomig, Maxalt, and Amerge. These drugs, like Ergot, can be dramatically effective in terminating the acute migraine attack.

A variety of agents have been used as prophylactics for the prevention of migraine. Sansert was the first. Inderal, a noradrenaline blocking agent, was the second. The tricyclics have long been used in the prevention of migraine (they don't really work very well, though). Lithium is occasionally effective, and the anticonvulsant drugs, Depakote, Topamax, and Neurontin, are also quite useful. This is usually the way it works in neuropsychiatric disease. A variety of greatly dissimilar drugs with different pharmacologic properties are effective in the treatment of a disease. As if we needed reminding, the brain is a complex place, and its disorders not given to simplistic understanding.

The remarkable advances in the treatment of migraine notwithstanding, we still don't really understand the disease. We don't know for sure whether its manifestations are due to erratic blood vessels, first constricted and then dilated, or to some kind of neural phenomenon independent of blood flow. There is absolutely no question that the pain of migraine can be relieved by giving vasoconstricting agents. The fact that these same drugs influence neurotransmitters which are present in the brain as well as the blood vessels is, however, certainly an annoying and confusing issue.

We tend to view migraine as an unfortunate, but in the long run, benign disease. Not always. Migraine occasionally produces injury and inflammation. Cerebral infarction, a stroke, can occur with migraine. Swelling and hemorrhage into the scalp and face are not uncommon. Sometimes the migraineur is left after an attack with a black eye. Paralysis of eye muscles with double vision and lid closure may accompany. A peculiar sort of inflammation occurs uniquely in cluster headaches. The disease is characterized by excruciating, rather brief unilateral eye and head pain associated with conjunctival suffusion. The surface of the eye is reddened, and the patient is unilaterally tearful. This effect can be vivid. The experienced clinician observing a person during an attack can make a diagnosis easily just by looking at him. Yes, him. Cluster, unlike most forms of migraine, occurs almost exclusively in the male.

Inflammation is the product of the body's response to noxious influence. This may be traumatic, infectious, neoplastic, or vascular. Is vascular disease the cause of bruising, extraocular muscle palsies, or red eyes when we have migraines? These occurrences, and they are seen with some frequency, are certainly in accord with the belief that migraine is a disease of blood vessels. There is, however, a body of evidence suggesting that migraine is the product of a neural rather than a vascular disorder. The phenomenon of spreading depression, a suppression of brain wave activity, occurs uniquely with migraine. It is never seen in cerebrovascular disease. Nor can the strange geometric hallucinations be ascribed to ischemia. They never occur with arteriosclerotic vascular disease, only migraine.

Is migraine a disease of blood vessels, or a disease of the nerves, or both? It continues to fascinate, but it still escapes understanding. Research into the issue, however, has offered a provocative discovery. That is the phenomenon of neurogenic inflammation, about which I have written before and will again soon.

Migraine is a French word, derived from the Greek, meaning pain on one half of the head. A singular attribute of migraine is its remarkable capacity for unilaterality. This is a hallmark and an identifier of the disease. Pain on one side sometimes, and sometimes on the other, and for sure, sometimes both. The visual and somatosensory effects of migraine are also unilateral and most of the time obey the rules of neuroanatomy. A left-sided headache predictably produces loss of vision to the right and numbness and weakness on the right, and occasionally disordered speech because that function resides in the left hemisphere. But migraine, unfathomable migraine, often defies even the most fundamental laws. Contrary to everything we know about brain function, a unilateral headache may be associated with loss of vision on the same side, a phenomenon that can only be understood by postulating that one half of the brain is producing pain and the other half visual loss—both sides misbehaving simultaneously in contrasting ways.

Curious that migraine, a disease without clear pathoanatomic correlates, should reflect itself so often in the form of laterality. Conceptually it staggers the imagination. Why should menstruating or eating Roquefort cheese produce pain in only one-half of the head? We can only marvel at our ignorance of the manner in which a fundamentally healthy brain disorganizes its function in such a bizarre manner. Perhaps it is because the subcortical brain, almost certainly the source of migraine, is so untopographic and unaware, unlike the cortical brain, of its leftness and rightness.

Migraine is an acutely painful experience, associated to be sure with a spectacular array of concomitants. As with every other painful experience, if life events dictate, it may not go away. The migraineur can, and often does, fail to recover. The result is the most common form of chronic pain.

Remember Christy with the median nerve injury. As a young woman she suffered migraine headaches. They were highly typical with peri-odic attacks of unilateral head pain followed by recovery. They were, at least early on, responsive to the drug Imitrex. Christy undoubtedly carried the genetic inheritance of migraine. She also very likely carried the genetic inheritance of depression. Whether this occurred by chance, for both are common diseases, or was the product of some biologic design is uncertain, but the two diseases, migraine and depression, certainly do seem to run in tandem. Christy entered her depression in her mid-twenties, several years after the onset of her migraines. As her depression evolved, she experienced a very common clinical phenomenon. Her headaches, formerly unilateral and periodic, became bilateral and incessant. The neural authority which dictated her migraine headaches was recon-figured by another authority, depression. Her headaches no longer responded to Imitrex. Nor did her depression respond to SSRIs. Her diseases had melded into another disorder, the syndrome of chronic pain. Her blue depression and her red-hot migraine were altered into a hybrid of another color, orange, and smoldering. A pain not so severe as migraine but more disturbing because it was incessant. Christy no longer had migraine, and she no longer experienced intervals of wellness. It was in this setting that she suffered an injury to her median nerve. She developed, and it is hard to imagine anything more predictable, relentless neuritic pain in the hand.

Treatments directed to her painfulness, in both the head and the hand, included the use of the neurotransmitter-altering agents, Imipramine, Klonopin, and Neurontin. Sleep and energy were restored, weight was lost, and painfulness, in both parts, was abated. Drug therapy resurrected remote routings to dominance and prior behaviors were restored. The reconfiguration was reconfigured. The latent behavior of wellness reappeared and with it, so did the latent behavior of migraine. As Christy got well, her headaches returned to their original structure, unilateral, pulsatile, and intermittent. To make the story complete, perfectly complete, they responded once again, as they had done years before, to Imitrex.

Migraine is not a free-standing entity. It is interrelated and comorbid with other diseases, and in the last analysis, subject to their persuasion. It could not be otherwise.

Christy had experienced, with her depression, the transformation of migraine into chronic headache. This evolution is well-recognized. What happened later, under drug therapy, the transformation of chronic headaches back into migraine is not so widely appreciated, and it should be. Many, indeed most neurologists, believe that tricyclic drugs are effective in the prevention of migraine. I don't think so. Just take a look at Christy. Her migraines reappeared during tricyclic therapy! Tricyclics are good for chronic pain. They are without peer in the treatment of that disease, but they are not good for migraine. Unfortunately, it is sometimes difficult to tell the difference between those diseases.

Migraine is a brain experience. It shares brain space and function with other experiences, those of thought and mood and the vegetative behaviors of sleep and appetite. Migraine is not a free-standing entity. It is interrelated and comorbid with other diseases, and in the last analysis, subject to their persuasion. It could not be otherwise.

Let's create a hypothetical patient, a female because migraine is predominant in that gender. Let's introduce a stressor, say the death of a loved one. In doing so, let's be aware that the stressor need not be nearly so dramatic. It may be trivial, perhaps some minor personal rejection, or it may even be indiscernible, perhaps some disruption of biologic rhythms. Regardless, our patient, genetically endowed with migraine, possesses a neural system readily available for exhibition. This is recruited—and quickly. The migraine machinery is there. No reconfiguration is necessary. With the appearance of stress, she experiences an increase in the frequency and severity of headache. This sudden worsening of migraine is a certain indicator that the infrastructure is being challenged. Our patient may recover spontaneously. Recovery is the rule, not the exception, as most of our brain's unravelings are transient experiences. If, however, we fail to recover, the subcortical brain, the mastermind of our behavior, disassembles into multiple expressions. This happens slowly. It takes time for the neural axis to reconfigure into maladaptive functioning, just as it takes time for drug therapy to reconfigure the axis into effective functioning.

Which maladaptation should appear first and which later is quite variable, but it usually begins with disordered sleep. As our patient suffers an increased frequency of her headaches, she will likely experience insomnia. Her appetite will change, perhaps with sweet cravings and weight gain or, on the other side of the scale (there is no way to predict), she will become anorectic. Mood will disfigure with despondency and apathy. Temperament will be disordered with anxiety and restlessness, and perhaps even mind-too-busy obsessions.

Migraine, now under the pervasive influence of other brain forces, loses its identity and transmogrifies into another state of illness. The characteristic spatial and temporal dimensions of headache change. Periodicity is lost. Pain is no longer occasional. It is constant. Its unilaterality disappears. Pain crosses the midline in a symmetrical and mirror image manner and becomes generalized. The exotic sensory effects, visual and otherwise, go away. No longer are there intervals of hemianopia or scotoma. They vanish, leaving only a trace of their legacy, the occasional appearance of vague scintillations in the periphery of the visual field. Our patient has transformed migraine, a hybrid, a mix of fragments and comorbidities—part depression, part migraine, and probably part a host of other derangements. Her pain no longer responds to anti-migraine drugs, and her depression does not respond to SSRIs. She doesn't have either of those diseases. She has chronic pain. And that disease responds rather predictably to the tricyclic drugs. These agents, as I surmised early on, are useful and perhaps exclusively useful in the sleep-disordered, and the most certain attribute of chronic pain is impaired sleep. It is a clear identifier of the disease. It is not an identifier of migraine. That disease, remember, is characterized by intervals of wellness, and wellness is not sleep-disturbed.

When, exactly, does migraine become chronic pain? It is quite impossible to say because it happens slowly and gradually. Nature does not draw straight lines in time or space. They are irregular, and curvilinear, and the evolution of migraine into chronic pain (or vice versa) does not occur at a precise point in time. Indeed, in the natural history of the diseases, and they both have a discernible natural history, their display may shift from predominant migraine for one interval and for another, chronic pain.

The distinction between migraine and chronic pain can challenge the resources of the most skillful physician. It is never simple. Perhaps our hypothetical patient is drinking too much. Substance abuse certainly weighs heavily in the scales. Perhaps our patient is bipolar, or perhaps she was abused in her youth. All these must be factored in. They invite the use of a variety of drugs for the treatment of a disease that we often presume to be migraine, but it is really not.

Transformed migraine is the disease that for so many years was, and unfortunately still is, misidentified as tension headaches—an egregious example of our proclivity to ascribe a state of pain to an inability to deal emotionally with the environment. Nothing really wrong with that, so long as we remember that many diseases are the product of inability to deal with the environment. No reason to single out headache for special treatment. We would hardly employ the phrases tension schizophrenia, or tension depression, or tension

heart attack. These are nonsensical because we recognize that each
of these disorders has a certain biologic substrate. We don't afford
headaches that dignity. It is too convenient to blame the patient.

Clinical medicine, as they say, is both art and science. Well, it used
to be. No longer. The astonishing ability to image the body and
understand the behavior of illness (undreamed of just a few decades
ago) has removed art from the practice of medicine and made it a
very scientific discipline. With science has come standardization.
We now have diagnostic protocols of elegant brevity and
simplicity. Those for migraine have been reduced to a page of
single-spaced copy. Unfortunately, in our quest for brevity and
coherence, making something simple out of that which is by no
means simple, we often miss the mark—and the diagnosis.

Janet was a proper, well-groomed, quiet, and unobtrusive woman. She was also
tightly bound, hesitant, and fearful of saying too much. There was
an air of suspicion and distrust. I could see that right away, and I
knew I was in for an interesting encounter.

She was experiencing headaches, moderate in severity and
frequent, occurring almost daily. They waxed and waned but never
quite went away. They were frontal in location and centered behind
her eyes and within her ears, radiating from these points to her
upper face and forehead and often into her jaws. They began a
couple of years before. An oral surgeon had advised surgical repair
of her temporomandibular joints, seemingly damaged by a remote
dental problem. Janet demurred and consulted her internist. He,
knowing Janet well, thought my evaluation might be in order.

Janet's attacks of pain lasted a few hours. They were bilateral
and pulsatile, and they were stereotyped. Her headaches were all
pretty much alike, uniform in their temporal and spatial display.
This stereotypy, the same pattern of recurrent headache, is almost
always an indicator of migraine. I began to dissect her descriptions
and asked a few pointed questions. Yes, she replied, sometimes her
vision was disordered during a headache. She would see little
sparkles on the edges of her vision, never in the center of it. They

were like little shining crystals. They lasted only a few minutes, her headaches much longer.

Stereotyped headaches, bilateral to be sure, but pulsatile and with visual scintillations and nausea. Certainly migraine, they met diagnostic criteria for the disease. It is never simple, however. I prodded Janet into more detailed descriptions. She was unaware, until we began exploring, that she actually had two types of headache. One was predominant in the face and the jaws, and the other in the eyes. She never experienced scintillations with jaw pain, but she almost invariably did with eye pain. Sure, both could still be migraine. There is no law of nature that says face and jaw pain can't be migraine. Its repetitive and stereotyped character, occurring in the patient whose other head pains were typical of migraine, is sufficient evidence to make a diagnosis of migraine for both.

I asked Janet whether she had ever experienced headaches in the past. She remembered them well. They happened twice when she was a teenager, and they were excruciating, with severe pain and vomiting. They lasted all day and put her in bed. After that she remained free of headaches for forty years.

I asked if she was sad or despondent. "Yes," she answered in the manner of so many painful patients, "I am depressed, but it is just because of the pain. You would be depressed too if you had these headaches."

"Do you sleep well?"

"No, I've never slept well. I can't sleep at all now. I can't get comfortable at night. The headache is always there. It keeps me awake. My bladder does too. I have to go to the bathroom three or four times."

"I am going to ask you a strange question. Do your legs ever bother you? Do they ever start jerking or moving uncontrollably?"

"How did you know that? At night when I go to bed, my legs are constantly moving. They are restless."

"How long have they been that way, and how long have you had trouble sleeping?"

"All my life, as far back as I can remember."

"Do you remember your childhood?"

"Yes, I remember it. It was horrible."

"Tell me about it."

"My father was alcoholic. He and my mother were always fighting. I watched him beat her many times."

"Were you ever beaten?"

"Yes, a couple times. Once he hit me in the face so hard that I lost my hearing. My jaw hurt for weeks after that."

She completed high school and found a job as a clerk in a government office. There she was to remain for forty years. She married and had a child. Then she entered, perhaps as a product of inheritance, alcoholism. Several years into it, Janet elected to enter a treatment center. A wonderful turn of events it would seem, but it was not to be. Drugs leave their mark. Life experiences leave their mark. Behavior and biology are inexorably intertwined, and the products of their alchemy can be quite unpredictable. With recovery Janet grew irascible, anxious, and depressed. She was hospitalized after a suicide attempt and was treated with Prozac, just arrived on the scene. It was very effective—Janet was restored to health.

Behavior and biology are inexorably intertwined, and the products of their alchemy can be quite unpredictable.

Several years later, on a routine dental visit, Janet was told that her teeth were eroding rapidly, the result of a dental malocclusion caused by a remotely fractured mandible. (Janet didn't tell her dentist about the beating.) Surgery to correct the problem was performed. Janet's jawbone was rebroken under anesthesia and restructured into more effective alignment. Following surgery, her jaw, even though immobilized by wiring, was excruciatingly painful. It took her a long time to recover, but she finally did, to continue her rather successful life, now elevated in the bureaucracy to an office of her own.

What stressor precipitated the illness that I was called upon to evaluate I do not know. None was evident in the history taking. Janet's life, considering how it started, had gone quite well. Now in her early maturity, her child and her husband doing well, she became painful in the head and the face. Sometimes we can clearly identify a precipitating stressor, but often we cannot. It may have been some chance encounter, or perhaps a disordered biologic rhythm, or an early cerebral involution. But something, we can be sure, precipitated a reconfiguration and the invocation of ancient memories and behaviors. Remote depression, a kindled experience was resurrected. Remote jaw pain also. Migraine, a years-removed childhood experience, was also gathered up and came along for the ride. Transformed they all were, melded together into the expression of a unique illness.

Janet was not an easy person to know or to treat. Suspicion and distrust are the legacy of childhood abuse. The physician must go gently and patiently. Negativism and self-defeating behaviors are common in depression and pain, especially so when they are generated by destructive childhood experiences. I prescribed Klonopin and Imipramine. I elected not to treat her with a specific anti-migraine drug such as Imitrex. I knew it wouldn't work, at least yet, and Janet didn't need failure at that stage of the game. She desperately needed some kind of success. I saw her two weeks later. I didn't expect her to be well, but I expected some improvement. I saw it very clearly, but distrustful Janet did not.

"I am just not sure about these drugs. I don't like drugs. I don't like being addicted."

"Janet, are you sleeping any better?"

"Yes, it is a little bit better. I don't get up quite as much."

"Do you feel any better? Do you have more energy?"

"No, I don't really feel any better. I don't like taking these drugs. I am not sure I really want to do this."

"Are your legs still restless?"

"No, they don't jerk so much."

"How about your pain, Janet? Are your headaches any different?"

"No! I don't like taking these drugs. My headaches are worse! I had a terrible headache a week ago. The worst one ever. It lasted all day."

"Did you have the sparkles with it?"

"I had more than sparkles. I could hardly see at all. There was a spot right in front of my eyes. It was white, and it had shining edges, and it got bigger and bigger until I couldn't see anything at all. I don't like these drugs."

"Janet, you said you had a real bad headache a week ago. Have you had other headaches?"

"No. That is the only headache I've had, but it was terrible."

"You only had one headache in the past two weeks. Is that correct? You told me you were having them every day."

"No, that was my only headache."

Janet was getting well, and the rapidity with which it was happening was really quite astonishing. In the course of a scant week or two, the structure of her neurobiology was changing. Her sleep was beginning to restore. Her nocturia and restless legs were abating, and her headaches dramatically changing in their clinical expression. Janet had just experienced a classic migraine headache, the first she had known since her teen years. I prescribed Imitrex should her headaches recur, and told her to increase the dosage of Imipramine. It didn't take long. Within another month Janet felt much better. It is amazing what wellness and trust can do. She was engaging, even flirtatous. The reconfiguration was reconfigured, and Janet's occasional migraines responded very well to Imitrex. She remains on Klonopin and Imipramine. Needful and appropriate polypharmacy for a disease that looks like migraine but is really not.

CHAPTER SEVENTEEN

Neurogenic Inflammation

M ac, retired from the insurance business, had a beautiful wife and an outstanding daughter. He also had migraine. Darvon gave him excellent relief, and he used the drug with some frequency, even to help him sleep at night. It was Mac's good fortune to have his disease well under control before the syndrome of analgesic rebound headache entered the diagnostic tables. Had Mac been withdrawn from his occasional use of Darvon, his life would have been, I am sure, much more complicated.

I attended Mac for many years. His migraine was never really an issue, at least until the day he called me to report an unusual event. He had just experienced one of his headaches and was already getting better with Darvon, but something very strange was happening to him. One of his eyelids was drooping, covering the pupil. Mac was able to see out of the eye only by manually lifting the lid.

Paralysis of the eyelid is usually due to damage to the third cranial nerve. It is often a sign of pressure on that nerve, most commonly due to an expanding aneurysm. I directed Mac to the emergency room, and a cerebral arteriogram to outline the brain's blood vessels was performed. There was no aneurysm. Thankful for that, I bedded Mac down for the night to observe the progress of his third nerve palsy. It occasionally occurs, partially or completely, with migraine, certainly a product of some kind of inflammation within the nerve.

The following morning, Mac had progressed to a total paralysis of eye movement. The globe was immobilized within the orbit,

169

unable to move right or left, up or down. Not only was the third nerve gone, but also the fourth and sixth! When the paralyzed lid was lifted, Mac's visual images were doubled, for the two eyes could no longer move in concert. Some time during the following night, Mac experienced a mirror image effect. When he awoke from sleep, the other eye was also paralyzed. When the lids were lifted, Mac could see without diplopia, for both eyes were stuck in the mid-position. He recovered in just a few days. Whether it was due to the cortisone I gave him, I am not sure.

The migrainous brain may have trouble deciding between its left and its right, but its ability to otherwise localize its malevolence is amazing. The selectivity of its inflammatory effects, directed in Mac exclusively to the nerves of eye movement, challenges credulity.

There are twelve cranial nerves, paired on each side. The first subserves the function of smell, the second of vision. The third, fourth, and sixth control eye movement. Between these, the fifth, the trigeminal nerve (the gasserian is its ganglion), serves the function of sensation in the face and head. Below are the nerves which control facial movement, audition, and the acts of swallowing and phonation. These nerves are in intimate juxtaposition within a very small space, the brain stem. Accordingly, a chance injury to the stem, such as a stroke or an attack of multiple sclerosis, almost always involves multiple nerves, partially or completely. The possibility of such an event, however, destroying the third, fourth, and sixth nerves exclusively, while sparing adjacent ones, is remote. To do so on both sides, virtually simultaneously, is well nigh impossible. The attack on Mac's nerves cannot be considered an accident, a chance event. It was directed and focused, exquisitely so, by authority.

Inherent to the function of vision is the symmetric and conjugate movement of the two eyes. The muscles of their movement, present on each side, are controlled by cells within the brain stem which integrate their actions. It was these cells, certainly, which directed the Mac attack. Like all brain cells, they are endowed with plasticity, the capacity to change their behavior. Subject to the malfeasance that is migraine, they directed their energy to the destruction of the nerves and muscles under their control. This brain-directed and highly localized inflammatory effect is known as neurogenic inflammation.

Most forms of inflammation, those caused by nociceptive injury, cut a wide swath. They pay little regard to tissue boundaries. They destroy whatever is in their way. A bony fracture will damage muscles, tendons, nerves, and blood vessels. An impacted gallstone will inflame the gallbladder and often also the contiguous liver and pancreas. Neurogenic inflammation, directed by brain authority, behaves quite differently. It is localized to a single body part. It does not spread to adjacent tissues. The unilaterally red eye of cluster headache, exquisitely localized to the conjunctiva, is an example. The Mac attack, the selective destruction of those cranial nerves dedicated to eye movement, was certainly a highly focused form of inflammation.

Neurogenic inflammation is by no means solely the province of migraine. Cerebral injury or drug intoxication incites neurogenic inflammation localized to the lungs' capillary bed, causing pulmonary edema. Cerebral injury can also damage the heart. Changes in the electrocardiogram, even those of a myocardial infarction, may occur in patients with stroke or intracranial hemorrhage. We know, with certainty, that the brain under provocation can damage, seemingly with great selectivity, the eyes, the heart, the lungs, and perhaps (remember Harriet) even the pericardium.

We know that somatic tissue is under neural control. When our tissues misbehave, as when we flush with embarrassment, or when our bowels are irritable, it is the product of neural stimulation. We all recognize this, but we have a little more difficulty recognizing that neural stimulation may actually produce injury and inflammation.

Sally was experiencing band-like pain around her chest. It began in the spine and radiated to the front—it was present bilaterally but worse on the left. It corresponded to the distribution of the fifth and sixth thoracic nerves. A spinal cord tumor or a herniated disc was suspect, but her neurosurgical work-up was normal in detail. Her diagnosis was intercostal neuritis, a vague entity indeed. It can certainly happen with shingles, but that disease, with its characteristic rash, is easy to diagnose. It can also occur with diabetes, but Sally did not have that disorder. There was no demonstrable pathology to account for her symptoms. I treated Sally with Doxepin.

She called a few days later to report some interesting developments. She was sleeping well, and her spirits had improved, but her pain was no better. I assured her that would likely come later, but she responded that she was unable to take the drug because she was allergic to it. She had developed a rash. She described it as little red spots on her chest but not elsewhere. This was suspicious. A drug rash is usually widespread. It may occasionally be localized, but I felt it was worth taking a look. I was surprised when I saw it. She had petchiae, evidence of small vessel hemorrhage, along the path of her fifth and sixth intercostal nerves. It was present on the left, more painful side, but not the right. Her rash followed the path of her painfulness, reaching from her back to her anterior chest. I was sure that this was not a drug reaction or shingles. It was, I believed then and believe now, a manifestation of neurogenic inflammation, hemorrhage along the path of pain, seemingly appearing under the aegis of my drug therapy.

Why should she experience such an untoward effect when she was clinically improving? Sometimes, even when we give the right drug, a drug that turns out to be successful in the long term, odd things happen at first. And why not? As we influence neurons, persuading them to reconfigure, they often along the way demonstrate transient maladaptions. The road to recovery is sometimes a bumpy road. I encouraged Sally to continue her therapy. Her rash and pain went away in just a few days.

I have had a personal experience with neurogenic inflammation. It was bizarre, trivial, and even amusing. It was also, I suspect, like most brain things, a product of memory. When I was a child I became ill with meningitis, and for a while it was a close go. During the course of my illness, I was in a coma for a few days and convulsive, and as my brain swelled with inflammation, my sixth cranial nerve was damaged and my eye crossed. I also hemorrhaged into my eyes and was, I am told, blind for several days. I have no recollection at all of the event, but somewhere, I am sure, hidden in the recesses of my mind, is a memory of childhood illness and visual loss. This may be the reason I am so sensitive, even phobic, about my eyes. This has always been a bit of a problem, and I do not enjoy my visits to the ophthalmologist.

On one of my eye exams, I requested to be fitted for contact lenses. The best way to cure a phobia, after all, is to attack it directly and head on. The ophthalmologist began the refraction exercises by darkening the room and then illuminating a screen with a series of letters. As he introduced in rapid succession a variety of lenses to alter my acuity, I responded with each change whether my vision was better or worse. In my efforts to be precise, and at the same time cooperative and accommodating, I gave inconsistent answers. My doctor could not, to his satisfaction, obtain a reproducible response. Nothing to do but keep repeating the exercises until there was consistency. I was subjected to repeated flashes of light, *stroboscopic stimulation*. The stimulus is often employed in electroencephalography in an attempt to provoke epileptic activity. Flashing lights can certainly precipitate a seizure. They did in me. I slumped forward, jerked my arms a few times, and then woke up. It wasn't much of a convulsion. It might even have represented a *vasovagal* effect. That is a form of dysautonomia, a sudden slowing of the heart rate or loss of blood pressure that occurs with noxious stimulation. I suspect, however, that it was an epileptic seizure. After all, I had had one before under the provocation of meningitis. Perhaps a remote memory recrudesced under stroboscopic stimulation. I was well in just a few moments, less frightened than humiliated and embarrassed by the experience.

My own response to the event was, in the last analysis, a form of denial. I really didn't want to submit myself to an MRI and electroencephalogram. This was not an unsound clinical judgment at all. Single seizures sometimes occur in extenuating circumstances and do not warrant a diagnosis of epilepsy. So I entered denial, trying to repress a threatening memory. It was not, however, to be forgotten. It remained to reinforce my ongoing fear of ophthalmologists and their examining suites.

Some years later, I noticed that when I rubbed my eyes, I would displace one of my contact lenses. It happened repetitively, but I paid it no attention until a friend pointed out that I had a lump on my upper eyelid. I had developed a chalazion, a cyst in the lid. Hardly a bother, it was barely noticeable, at least until one knew it was there. I resolved to have it removed. Again, overcome your phobias by attacking them—but not too hard. A return to the site of my humiliation was more than I wanted to bear, so I went to a different ophthalmologist.

"You have a chalazion," he said.

"Yes, and I would like for you to remove it for me."

"We really don't have to do anything about it. It is not bothering you, and it doesn't look bad."

"I'm sorry, but it does bother me. I would appreciate your removing it."

"Okay." He led me to his operating suite. I heard his sigh.

"Do you ever get vasovagal?"

"Yes, I am somewhat subject to that, but I don't think it will be a problem." I didn't tell him about my convulsion.

Manipulation of the eyes frequently slows the heart rate by stimulating the vagus nerve. Indeed, in times remote, we used to try to arrest tachycardia by applying pressure to the eyes. I began to suspect that my physician had seen enough faints with eyelid surgery to not be very enthusiastic about performing the operation. This reinforced my already considerable anxiety. Nonetheless, I affected comfort and nonchalance. I was anything but. As I positioned myself for surgery, I placed my hands across my lap, the fingers of one on the radial artery of the other to measure my autonomic response to an experience that I was dreading.

The brain consumes an enormous share of the body's metabolic energy. Billions of active cells, employing glucose as their life force, use it at prodigious rates, even at rest. Supine and immobilized, I was hardly at rest. My anxieties and fears were mounting, and I was employing reserves of energy to control them. A fearful and humiliating memory of a convulsive seizure possessed my awareness. What would happen, I did not know. Perhaps a faint. Perhaps even a convulsion. Nothing to do but wait it out and hope for the best. I don't know what good counting my pulse did for me, but at least it was a distraction.

Then the surgical lamp. An intense bright light four feet from my face! Another stimulus, another memory.

"I am sorry, but this is going to hurt a little bit." He introduced a needle into my upper eyelid, and the nerves of that richly innervated structure were traumatized by penetration and the introduction of an anesthetic and with it, tissue distention and stretch. Painful it was. A message entered my trigeminal nerve and from there to the gasserian ganglion where it was relayed through my analgesic centers and then throughout my subcortical brain, insinuating itself and recruiting a host of memories on its way to the thalamus and conscious perception. Still, seventy-two and steady.

The ophthalmologist placed a clamp with an oval window on my eyelid and everted the structure, exposing the inside to the outside. Painless with anesthetic, I felt no discomfort as the cyst was incised and the foreign material curetted out. It was all over in just a few moments. I arose slowly, fearing a faint, but it did not occur.

"It looked like there was a little infection in there, so I am giving you an antibiotic to put on your lid a couple of times a day. There is no need for follow-up. I don't need to see you until you develop another one," he joked. I laughed too. There is nothing quite so beautiful as the satisfactory completion of a stressful task. That evening I studied my surgeon's handiwork and was pleased. The cyst was gone and my eye unblemished.

The following morning I looked in the mirror to apply the antibiotic ointment. I had to look twice—three times—to believe what I was seeing. When I went to bed the night before, my eye was normal in appearance. Hours later, there was an oval area of hemorrhage conforming exactly to the dimensions of the clamp he had placed the day before. The hemorrhage, however, was on my left upper eyelid. He had operated on the right! The left had not been touched.

It was a bizarre and strange, but by no means unaccountable, occurrence. The bizarre happens quite a lot in clinical medicine. We usually ascribe it to coincidence, but by no stretch of the imagination was my left eye hemorrhage unrelated to my right eye operation. No way it could have been. The lesion was exquisitely focused and brain-directed, an example of neurogenic inflammation, albeit one with misdirected laterality.

During the interval of my minor surgery, I was under great stress, my slow and steady pulse notwithstanding. My cerebral apparatus was disarrayed and in conflict, this generated by a variety of experiences. There certainly were plenty to choose from. Childhood meningitis with convulsions and blindness, fear of ophthalmologists, exposure to a very bright light and the disturbing memories that it entailed, and the experience of severe pain in my right eye. Were these operative in my brain's curious and transient misbehavior? My neurogenic inflammation did not occur immediately after surgery. It happened later, when I was asleep. Is that a coincidence? Probably not. Sleep is a potent activator of brain misbehavior. Flashbacks, restless legs, and many forms of pain appear under the provocation of sleep. Could not neurogenic inflammation also?

To top it all off, there was an exquisite fillip, this in the form of left-right brain confusion. The subcortical brain has limited topographic ability. Although it can sometimes direct its energy to well-localized placement in the body, it has inordinate difficulty with laterality. My pain went in on the right, and the neurogenic response came out on the left.

Subcortical neurons are plastic, and they have the capacity for choice—and surprise. Our neural routings are not one-way streets. They are bidirectional, and sometimes the electrochemical message does not go the way it should. The referral of pain, the perception of its originating away from the site of injury, is an example of misdirection. And so is neurogenic inflammation. A message in the form of a painful signal enters the brain and reflexly goes back down to incite inflammation. This is what happened to Mac's eye muscles, to Sally's thoracic nerves, to my eyelid, and to Harriet's pericardium. It is also what happens in reflex sympathetic dystrophy. As the very name of the disorder implies, the brain in response to pain reflexly attacks the body.

I have written of the many strange clinical expressions of chronic pain, and neurogenic inflammation is certainly the strangest. Bizarre though it is, it just may help us understand the behavior of some common disorders. Is it possible that inflammatory diseases, such as arthritis, could actually be generated by messages from the brain? The suggestion that a disordered mind could actually inflame the joints borders on the ludicrous, but it probably does happen.

Erich was an auto mechanic. An operation to fuse his unstable cervical vertebrae and relieve his chronic neck and arm pain had been performed a year before. It was unsuccessful. He entered a sleepless depression and began to experience burning pain in his hands. Another surgery, to repair a damaged carpal tunnel, was performed but this, too, was unsuccessful. I saw him on referral and recorded his medical history. He had experienced depression along the way throughout his life, and also arthritic knees. They were frequently swollen, stiff, and painful. His orthopedist treated him with periodic injections of cortisone. This procedure was performed every three months, the maximum frequency allowed. Following each injection, pain would temper, and mobility would be restored for several weeks. This had gone on for three or four years.

I directed my attention to the neck and hand pain, prescribing Imipramine and Klonopin. Their performance was spotty. Sleep and depression improved substantially and neck pain was diminished, but hand pain continued. It remained even after a second operation to explore the carpal tunnel. A couple of years into

> *I have written of the many strange clinical expressions of chronic pain, and neurogenic inflammation is certainly the strangest. Bizarre though it is, it just may help us understand the behavior of some common disorders.*

treatment, after trials of many drugs, I told Erich that I had nothing more to offer. He would just have to live with his hand pain. He expressed appreciation for my efforts and told me that he was not unhappy with the outcome. His neck pain and his depression were relieved, and his arthritic joints no longer bothered him. From the day I gave him Imipramine and Klonopin, Erich never experienced knee pain or swelling again. He had not required a cortisone injection for two years.

In wellness, the painful message from an arthritic joint is modulated and controlled, at least partially, by the brain's analgesic systems. In those patients whose cerebral function is disarrayed by depression, substance abuse, or any of the other comorbidities which incite chronic pain, however, the message can be mishandled and sent back down in the form of neurogenic inflammation. Some day, probably in the not distant future, we will accept the use of mind drugs in the treatment of inflammatory disease. In a sense, we already do this when we treat migraine.

CHAPTER EIGHTEEN

Attention Deficit Disorder

Keith was short and round. His face was unlined, but his countenance was one of resignation. In the course of the preliminaries, I inquired about his family and his work. His ancestry, he told me, was distinguished. "I would have been rich, but the family fought, and my father was on the losing side."

"You certainly live in a nice part of town. You must have done rather well."

"I did okay. I was a banker, and I had some success, but not as much as I should have."

"Why is that?"

"I hate to say it, but I am not very smart. My grades in school were terrible. I didn't test well because it took me too long to organize my thoughts. That was my problem in banking. It took me forever to assemble a loan statement."

In a few short moments, I had learned quite a lot about my patient—even before we addressed the clinical details. Eight years before, an arthritic knee was replaced. Mobility was restored, but pain continued. Then, a ruptured lumbar disc with back and leg pain. The disc was surgically removed, but pain remained. A couple of years later, a fall on the ice and a hip fracture. The joint was repaired, but Keith failed to recover from that operation also. He remained painful in his knee, back, and hip, and as predictably happens, pain spread to other body parts. Eight years into his illness, he was total body painful. He saw many doctors and with each consultation, he told me, he acquired another diagnosis—tendonitis, fibromyalgia, carpal tunnel syndrome, and heel spurs.

He was given opiates, first Hydrocodone, and then Duragesic patches, 50 micrograms every third day. He was also given Prozac which he found unhelpful.

He brought with him, as painful patients often do, a summary of his medical adventures and misadventures. A decade of his life transcribed onto two pages. Painful patients are often compulsive record keepers. These notes can be very helpful. The hard data is available for easy access. Time can be spent on more important things.

In our maturity, and sometimes before, our bodies start to fall apart. The random appearance of fractured hips, ruptured discs, and arthritic knees are the chance signs of our decay. In Keith's case, however, the incredible sequence of failure to recover could not be ascribed to chance. It was certainly appearing under authority, but what?

He denied any history of depression. I asked if he had ever experienced intervals of euphoria or empowerment. "No," he replied, "I've always been pretty even, never too good, never too bad."

"Do you drink, Keith? Have you ever had a problem with drugs?"

"A couple of glasses of wine every day, that's all."

"You made references to your childhood and your problems in school. Did you ever feel that you were mistreated or neglected?"

"No, my parents were good to me. I was just a lousy student."

I could find no antecedents for Keith's painfulness. Why it should appear so destructively late in his life was not apparent. I continued my history taking and obtained a curious bit of information. Throughout his life, Keith had been weight-irregular. He would periodically lose his appetite and shed twenty or thirty pounds, only to regain it gradually over the course of several weeks. There was no binge eating or purging. There was no particular emotional content to his weight loss or gain. It occurred whether he was glad or sad. It happened several times through his life, and he was quite unable to explain why.

A history of unaccountable weight fluctuation is common in the painful patient, just as is a history of disordered sleep. Keith's sleep, however, had never really been disturbed until the advent of his painfulness and even then, it was restored very satisfactorily with

Ambien. In most painful patients there are discernible antecedents. Keith's were modest. Disordered appetite and a life of unfulfillment. Not much to go on.

I prescribed Klonopin and Imipramine and told him to discard Ambien. He would, for the time being, continue Prozac and the opiate patches. On his return visit a couple of weeks later, he reported that he felt a little more positive and hopeful, but that his pain was unchanged. I advised him that it takes a while for the drugs to start working and instructed him to increase his dose of Imipramine. Anticipating that his pain might diminish, I wrote a prescription for a 25 rather than a 50 microgram Duragesic patch. I told him to see if he could get by on the smaller dose, but if that was inadequate, he could simply apply a second patch of 25 micrograms, giving him the equal of the 50 he had been accustomed to.

"You don't want me to take the Ambien, do you?"

"No, Keith, you stopped the Ambien two weeks ago, didn't you?"

"Yes, I am pretty sure I stopped that. I am taking a little orange pill at bedtime. What is that?"

"If you are just taking one of them, Keith, it should be Klonopin. You really should learn the names of these medicines. It is hard to identify them by their color."

"And the other pills, what is their name?"

"That should be Imipramine, and you are supposed to be taking three of them. The instructions are on the bottle. How many are you taking, and do you take them all at bedtime?"

"Yes, those are the green ones. I am not sure. I think I take one or two a day."

"At bedtime?"

"Yes, I take them all at bedtime. You told me to take the Prozac at bedtime too, didn't you?"

"Not really, Keith. I don't care when you take your Prozac. You can take that at the same time you were taking it before you came to me."

"Now, what about those patches? I have been using one, and now you want me to use two. Are you increasing the dose? I sure hope so. I need more pain relief."

"No, Keith. I am trying to decrease the dose. See if you can get by on one instead of two."

The conversation was frustrating to me, but Keith evidenced no frustration at all. He was, it seemed, quite comfortable with his inability to collect his thoughts. He was used to it.

Attention deficit disorder can occur in the adult, of that there is no doubt. But the diagnosis of ADD in a sixty-year-old is suspect—highly suspect. Nonetheless, there are psychiatrists (a few anyway) who treat the inattention and disorganized thought of the elderly with Ritalin. Sometimes it works. In Keith's case, the diagnosis of attention deficit disorder was not that unseemly. His poor academic performance and his lifelong inability to organize his thoughts, whether in banking or counting pills, was a clue. In the treatment of the painful, every clue is important, even if we have to bend the diagnostic tables a bit.

"I do like that Ritalin. I can think better. I am more focused now."

"Is it keeping you from sleeping?"

"No, I sleep even better now, and I feel better when I wake up."

"How about your pain, Keith? Is your pain any different?"

"Yes, it is a little better. Maybe it is an eight now where it used to be a ten. I'm using the little patch. It seems to be working."

I pushed the Imipramine dose up, but not by much. The drug slows the bladder, and many sixty-year-old males have slow bladders anyway. Keith settled down for the long haul on Imipramine, Klonopin, Ritalin, and Duragesic, waiting for time, the ally of the painful, to exert its influence. Will Keith get well? Almost certainly not. He will get better, but not well. His painfulness had been kindled for nearly a decade. It won't be easily chased away.

Keith's repeated failure to recover was not the product of chance. It was almost certainly dictated by authority. Was it the same authority that dictated his difficulty with thought? Would Keith have been a better student and better banker if he had received Ritalin along the way? Would he have been so painful?

Keith didn't really fulfill the diagnostic criteria for ADD, but he probably had some fragment of the disorder. This may be an unscientific judgment, but it is hardly an unworthy one. Psychiatric illnesses frequently appear in partials and *formes fruste*, and these fragments, as

I have certainly tried to emphasize, may coexist with chronic pain. Recognition of this association often leads the physician to effective (and even rational) therapy.

I will now abandon the narrative form and present a patient's intake history, written by her, and then my own office notes. Both were done under the press of time without regard to grammatical correctness. They convey a sense of immediacy as the patient talks to the doctor, and the doctor talks to himself.

Patient: Sue Jones

Date: 12/12/01

Ht: 5'4   Wt: 136   Temp: 98⁶
BP: 130 / 78   Pulse: 72

HISTORY

CHIEF COMPLAINT: Fibromyligia

HISTORY of PRESENT ILLNESS:

- Location: migraines / Neck Pain   • Quality

- Severity: Intense / debilitating /chemical   • Duration: Lst. Tuesday – Friday

- Timing: Yes/weather changes, Sensitivities RAIN   Context: Work, smell perfume + weather cgs.

- Associated signs/symptoms: Neck pain, base of scull, Insomnia, Lack of concentration Fatigue   • Modifying factors: Yes, previous episodes since I was 19 - better lay down, heat, cold, walk

  Bette - massage, hot shower medication /sleep

MEDICAL HISTORY:

- Patient medical history

	No	Yes
Diabetes	(No)	Yes
Hypertension	(No)	Yes
Cancer	No	(Yes)
Stroke	(No)	Yes
Heart trouble	(No)	Yes
Arthritis/gout	No	(Yes) osteo
Convulsions	(No)	Yes
Bleeding tendency	(No)	Yes
Acute infections	No	(Yes)
Venereal disease	(No)	Yes
Hereditary defects	No	(Yes)

Previous Hospitalizations/Surgeries/Serious Injuries   When?

Basal cell skin
Colonoscopy - irritable bowel

Medications (ocp) Luvox - Prozac -; (overall well being) Fiorcette, for migraine → Percocette, @ bed. / ambien

- Patient social history

Marital status: Single___ Married ✓ Separated___ Divorced___ Widowed___
Use of alcohol: Never ✓ Rarely___ Moderate___ Daily___
Use of tobacco: Never___ Previously, but quit___ Current packs/day Closet smoking 5-10 cigs per day
Use of drugs: Never ✓ Type/Frequency
Excessive exposure at home or work to: Fumes___ Dust___ Solvents___ Air-borne particles___ Noise___

December 12, 2001

Sue Jones—thirty-five years old—long interview with this lady, quite long. She found me through a friend who referred her. She carries a diagnosis of fibromyalgia. She has the whole nine yards. There was repeated childhood abuse. Father was erratic behavior and alcoholic. Died recently. They were estranged. She is also estranged from her mother. Been married a couple of times, one child, and depression early on. Diagnosis of headaches, migraine and otherwise, and irritable bowel syndrome. Married at age eighteen to get away. Had her child at age nineteen. Depressed throughout most of her life, maybe some hypomanic behavior. A lot of emotional illness in the family, and one sister suspected to be bipolar. She does data entry for an insurance company.

Given Prozac four years ago by her primary care doctor for PMS. She likes the drug and has stayed on it. Does have occasional bad headaches and was given some Percocet, but only occasionally for that. She does take Fioricet, probably on the order of two a day. It helps her chronic neck pain. Some three or four weeks ago, she was started on Luvox for suspect OCD. She does have some compulsive behaviors—a lot of hair-pulling and picking at her fingernails and cuticles. She can't tell if the Luvox has done anything yet. Long term sleepless—has taken many drugs, Ambien now.

Chronically fatigued, maybe some restless legs, description a little bit vague. Memory is impaired, sexual energy diminished. She is struggling to keep things on even keel. I think she has a chronic pain syndrome, ostensibly fibromyalgia, but also headaches, irritable bowels, and PMS—the whole nine yards with the usual antecedents. Tearful occasionally throughout our interview. She and I had a long talk, and I think she wants to work with me. I am going to have her stop the Luvox, continue the Prozac, and see what we can do with some Imipramine and Klonopin. Physical examination not remarkable. Heart and lungs clear. Animated, rapid speech, frightened, and frustrated. Two weeks.

December 27, 2001

Blood Pressure: 128/72   Weight: 134

Sue Jones returns, talking a blue streak. Brings a lot of reprints from fibromyalgia books for me to read. Comments that she is feeling better on the Imipramine 40 mg. and Klonopin 1 mg. than she has in quite a while. Sleep is better, nail and hair picking is better. Pain is diminishing, and she is actually having a reduction in appetite. She is excited about that. She is not having any real manic behavior, at least thus far. She is off the Luvox but remains on Prozac. Had more conversations about her illness and what it really means. She's somewhat insightful. She is now questioning whether she is bipolar. Perhaps, but that is on the back burner now. Regardless, she is happy with her progress. We will hold where we are now and take another look in a couple of weeks.

January 14, 2002

Blood Pressure: 124/74   Weight: 133

Sue Jones continues to do well. Not sleeping quite as well as she did before, but much more active, maybe too much. Went out and worked with her husband in the yard over the entire weekend. That was very pleasant. She has had some encounters with her mother and that has been unpleasant. She is thinking about renewing counseling. I think that is a fine idea. I gave her Dr. Smith's name. She can pursue that if she wishes. A little dry mouth, but no other problems with Imipramine. I am going to try and increase that from 40 up to 60. She came in a little bit early for refills because she is going out of town. Pretty good progress thus far. Her OCD behaviors, her toenail and fingernail and hair picking are much improved. She can actually wear open toe shoes and keep polish on the toenails and fingernails. Three weeks.

February 6, 2002

Blood Pressure: 130/70   Weight: 131

Not quite sustaining her improvement. Still better than we were by a long shot. Got the Imipramine up to 60 mg. I am going to move that up to 100 mg. and start her on some Topamax 25 mg.

daily for a week, then twice daily. Take another look in three weeks.
A lot good is happening, although some of her obsessive behaviors
are returning now and maybe a little bit of the pain. She certainly
is wired—incessant speech.

February 28, 2002

        Blood Pressure: 120/72   *Weight: 130*

    Not going to tolerate Topomax. Developed severe pain in the
gums after starting it—also depressed, forgetful, cross, and irritable.
Also flashbacks and some thoughts of suicide. Stop Topomax!! It is
not the drug for her. I am going to get that out of her system, then
try a little Ritalin. This could be ADD. Ritalin 10 mg., 1 to 2 a day,
continue the Imipramine, Klonopin, and Prozac. Two weeks.

March 13, 2002

        Blood Pressure: 124/70   *Weight: 129*

    Vast improvement! Fibromyalgia pain much diminished. No
headaches. No diarrhea. Compulsive nail picking almost totally
gone. Continues to lose weight and very happy about it. Blood
pressure okay, no adverse effects from Ritalin. She needs more.
Increase to 40 mg. daily. Said I should be able to tell she is better
because she no longer interrupts me whenever I speak. Says everything is better—more controlled—can think better. ADD it
probably is. OCD also.

A marvelous outcome—one of the best ever! In the span of but a
few weeks, the pain of fibromyalgia, irritable bowels, and headache
disappeared. Mood was lifted, compulsions arrested, and thought
reformed. Unnecessary weight was lost and necessary energy and
sleep restored. Did I not write, early on, that the experience of pain
cannot be separated form the experiences of thought, mood, sleep,
and appetite? And memory also. Sue was subject to the most
distressing of memories, that of sexual abuse at the hands of her
father.

    Will Sue stay well? Perhaps not. Her disease is subject to the
persuasion of unforeseeable forces, be these destructive life events,

shifts in biologic rhythms, or the intercurrence of other diseases. She will suffer relapses, and she will also suffer, along the way, side effects of her drugs. But, and this bears emphasis, so will patients with diabetes, hypertension, and arthritis. Sue will handle her reverses well, however, just as do most patients with the so-called organic diseases, because, like them, she now has some under-standing of the true meaning of her illness. She has felt the magic of the drugs. She is armed with knowledge—and hope. It is the lack of hope that most defines the illness, chronic pain. And it is the acquisition of hope that most certainly heralds recovery. Reverses there will be for sure, but there is great probability that the last half of Sue's life will be vastly more comfortable than the first.

Sue Jones's treatment was an absolutely brilliant exercise in polypharmacy. It was, I assure the reader, not only the product of skill but also of persistence. I didn't really find the drugs which fit the patient. Luckily, I just happened to find a patient who fit the drugs. A subtle distinction, perhaps, but not a bad way of looking at it. Regardless, the drugs worked and astonishingly well. Why did I succeed when other physicians, certainly of equal competence, did not? Was her improvement predicated on my telling her at the beginning that I thought there were drugs which might help her? Was my behavior so commanding and so hopeful that her response to my therapy represented a mere placebo effect? Discard that notion immediately! It is no placebo effect when the blood sugar falls in response to drug therapy, nor is it a placebo effect when the heart swollen with congestion responds to drug therapy. Nor is it when pain diminishes. Much as I might enjoy believing it, it is not the physician that cures chronic pain, it is the drugs.

Let's explore her treatment in a little detail. The reader is advised that my judgments are personal and admittedly opinionated. Nonetheless, they were successful, so they are probably worth paying attention to. Sue had seen many doctors before she came to me. Their choice of drugs, Ambien for sleep, Prozac for depression and the premenstrual syndrome, Luvox for obsessive-compulsive disorder, and Percocet and Fioricet for pain were certainly appro-priate, but in the last analysis, they were ineffective. Her physicians had treated the pieces, not the whole. So much for the diagnostic tables. They actually can be very destructive. During the course of her illness, Sue had never been treated with a tricyclic drug. They are old-fashioned, and often considered unworthy compared to the more refined contemporary pharmacy. Nonetheless, they remain the bedrock of the treatment of chronic pain. They do have significant side effects. Sedation, dry mouth, and sexual dsyfunction occur commonly, but the most dramatic and fearful side effect is the induction of mania. That possibility must remain in the mind of the physician because one of the epicenters of chronic pain, surely, is that of bipolar disease. Nonetheless, I prescribed a tricyclic, Imipramine, and also Klonopin, which I believe to be helpful in the treatment of pain. The downside to that drug is the risk of addiction. It's also an inherent risk in the use of opiates, but if the physician's treatment choices are guided by the fear of addiction, the physician should get out of the pain business.

Sue's response was almost immediate. Her many pains diminished. Her depression ameliorated. Her sleep came back and so did the pleasure of applying nail polish. Luvox, the right drug for obsessive-compulsive disorder, had not worked, but Imipramine did. Not really a surprise—Anafranil, a tricyclic similar to Imipramine, is often used for OCD. It is right up there with Luvox as a first choice. Once again, the right drug is the drug which works, and Imipramine certainly did that, in spades.

Success to be sure, but maybe also a warning. With her recovery, Sue was energized. She enjoyed cleaning her house and gardening to an extent she had never known before. She was happy and empowered. Was Sue entering mania? An incredible sense of well being often comes to those who recover from illness. This *flight to health* is common in those who are entering recovery from drug addiction. It is also common in those who enter recovery from chronic pain. It is certainly an understandable behavior in that disease, but occasionally it represents the unleashing of mania by tricyclic therapy. Sue's behaviors were almost manic. Not only was she energized in her physical acts, but also in her speech. It was rapid and discursive, with frequent arrests and shifts from one thought pattern to another. Was Sue bipolar? I suspected that she might be, and for that reason I chose Topamax. It is a good drug for mania, as well as pain, and all considered, a worthy addition to tricyclic and benzodiazepine therapy. She suffered dreadful side effects. Other epicenters, deep within the recesses of her mind and her memory, were intruded upon and provoked into exhibition. Pain, which had been diminishing from her head, her shoulders, and her belly was reincarnated into, of all places, her gums. Remote experiences were resurrected with frightening flashbacks. Temperament was altered with fractiousness and aggressiveness, and an obsessive thought, that of ending of her life, pervaded her consciousness. It can happen, and it does happen, not just with Topamax, but with Imipramine and Prozac and any other drug we use for the treatment of the mind-soul. Risk is inherent in the administration of any drug, but more so, I believe, in the treatment of chronic pain than any other disease—a reflection again of its complexity and the variety of neural mechanisms that enter its generation. Looking at it that way, we should expect more strange side effects in the treatment of chronic pain than any other disease, and unfortunately, we often get them.

> *Risk is inherent in the administration of any drug, but more so, I believe, in the treatment of chronic pain than any other disease . . .*

Sue recognized quickly that she was on a bad drug trip and with termination of that drug, she returned abruptly to her prior state of near-wellness, but she continued to talk incessantly. She constantly interrupted, and she could not sustain conversation. Mania it probably was not, but attention deficit disorder it certainly could have been. I chose Ritalin and it worked. Another epicenter was tempered. The ability to organize thought and speech was restored. As they fell under control, so, almost completely, did pain, depression, and compulsions.

Many physicians are beginning to suspect that attention deficit disorder and bipolar disease are one in the same illness. Both are attended by thought-racing, restless hyperactivity, interludes of depression, and, I suggest, chronic pain. Mental illnesses often change their display along the dimension of time (in much the same manner that chronic pain changes its display). Thus, attention-deprived, Ritalin-responsive hyperactivity in youth and manic, Lithium-responsive hyperactivity in adulthood (and sometimes, surely, it works the other way around).

The case histories presented in this book may appear to represent extraordinary examples of chronic pain, but they are not. They are very representative cases. In the great majority of painful patients, the origins of the disease can be traced to destructive life experiences, be these emotional, physical, or pharmacologic, or to psychiatric comorbidities. It usually can be traced to both, for destructive life experiences and psychiatric disease certainly march hand in hand. I will admit that I do occasionally see patients with chronic pain who do not suffer identifiable psychiatric illness and whose lives, in the main, have been contented and successful. I also occasionally see lung cancer in people who have never smoked. Draw your own conclusions.

I have described patients with a variety of painful diseases. In each of these I have, by dissecting their medical and personal histories and analyzing their response to drugs, pointed out their association with an equal variety of psychiatric disorders. Is this merely coincidence? Chronic pain, in its many forms, is a very common disease. Therefore, the chance concurrence of other, unrelated diseases is to be expected. While few physicians knowledgeable in matters painful would deny an association between chronic pain and depression, drug dependency, and childhood abuse, the association with the less common psychiatric disorders of bipolar disease, post-traumatic stress disorder, attention deficit disorder, and obsessive-compulsive disorder is much less certain. Their connection with chronic pain would probably not withstand statistical challenge. Nonetheless, I suspect it's there.

Chronic pain is not a disorder of spirit. It is a disorder of the mind's biology. It is the product of the abnormal release and uptake of neurotransmitting chemicals, and it obeys the commands of the same laws of biology that dictate the behavior of depression, bipolar disease, and all the rest. Unpleasant though this judgment may be, it is the most hopeful observation that we can offer about chronic pain, for when medical science finally finds the cure for the mental illnesses, and with pharmacy it is well on the way, it will surely have found the cure for chronic pain.

·

CHAPTER NINETEEN

Summing Up

I have attended many painful patients, most of whom have been sick for many months and often many years. They have defied conventional, and often unconventional, treatments. What is their recovery rate? It's over 50 percent, a lot better than it was just a few years ago. Even at best, however, recovery is incomplete. Ongoing drug therapy is necessary, just as it is necessary in diabetes and hypertension. Nonetheless, amelioration of pain sufficient for a life of relative comfort can be achieved.

Why do patients get better? It is the drugs. Without question, it is the drugs. If they are so good, why don't more people recover? The reasons are three. They are the comorbidities of opiate dependency, the devastation imposed by childhood abuse, and—perhaps most importantly—our societal and medical attitudes toward the disease, chronic pain.

In painfulness, as in no other illness, the effort to recover is balanced unfavorably by the effort to achieve other satisfactions. This is the conundrum of opiate therapy. Compassionate in usage, it nevertheless destroys those brain mechanisms which could sponsor recovery. With opiate therapy, the brain's analgesic systems wither and atrophy. (This declaration has no scientific proof, but nearly everyone suspects that it happens.) Opiate therapy deprives the patient not only of the psychologic resources for recovery, but also the physiologic resources.

We do a poor job of treating painfulness and the comorbidity of opiate dependency because we often employ blame as a treatment strategy. "If you will just stop taking those pills, your headache will get better." We blame the patient, and that is not a very useful modality in the treatment of substance abuse. We used to blame the alcoholic for his disease. It was only when we discarded the idea that alcoholism was due to characterologic weakness that we achieved any hope of meaningful recovery.

Over half of the patients that I see are on opiate therapy, most over many years. The recovery rate in this group is very low, just as the recovery rate in the treatment of depression associated with drug abuse is low. Only when we have treatment centers and a coherent strategy of pharmacologic and non-pharmacologic therapies will we ever achieve any significant cure of painfulness and its comorbidity, substance abuse. To create these centers and support them would be enormously expensive—but less expensive than the multiple-doctor, multiple-test, multiple-operation, and multiple-failure system that we now support.

The role of childhood abuse in the creation of the painful state must once again be addressed. The incidence of that experience in those who suffer chronic pain is staggeringly high. The occurrence of painfulness as a product of abuse, particularly sexual abuse, could almost certainly be diminished by early recognition, intervention, and care, but the event is usually entered into denial, there to kindle into chronic pain. I am inexpert in the modes of counseling and psychiatric care of the sexually abused, but I will offer a judgment. Treatments are directed to removing the patient from guilt and shame. This is a laudable and worthy aspiration, just as it is in the treatment of substance abuse. Nonetheless, I often see women who have completed their counseling, come to grips with their experience, and addressed their perpetrator with purpose, finality, and a sense of worth. Guilt is removed, but the pain goes on. We do not yet understand how to handle these patients. Drug therapy, for reasons already mentioned, is often not very effective.

We will not cure the painfulness of substance dependency or childhood abuse without restructuring our treatment protocols. Nor will we cure more than 50 percent of painful patients without restructuring our societal attitudes toward their disease.

An astonishing fact. At least a third of my painful patients have had to retain an attorney to seek redress for grievances and even to obtain, under Workers' Compensation, proper medical care. They bring suits against insurance companies, employers, and not infrequently, physicians. They require legal aid in obtaining disability and Social Security benefits. What would be the treatment outcomes in congestive heart failure or diabetes if a third of those patients were in litigation because of their disease?

We employ incredible technology in the care of the sick. The most important form of medical technology is the machine which images. Whether by computerized axial tomography, magnetic resonance imaging, or angiography, it rules the medical universe. It is our God. We are its servants, and as such, we have endowed our God with the attribute of omnipotence (which it very nearly deserves). When God tells us what is wrong with the patient, we are accepting. However, when God tell us that nothing is wrong with the patient, we are also accepting. A God of infinite power can also be a God of retribution.

Georgia hurt all the way from her low back to her neck. Her orthopedist performed an MRI. It was normal, nary a thing out of place. She was in her late thirties and wore a pullover with the words "Jesus Saves" across the front of it. She was obsessive about her pain and the destruction it had wrought in her life. She was the mother of two and, until her injury, a waitress at a truck stop. She fell while working there and experienced pain which didn't go away. She was unable to return to work. Her faith would carry her through this thing, she told me, just as it would carry her through her divorce. Her husband had left her just a few months before the accident, and he was not timely in his child support. Her examination was unremarkable, save for her painful behaviors, with stiffness, limping, and grimacing.

"God will help me. I know He will, but I need your assistance."

I told her I would try, but I knew it wouldn't be easy. She was already in litigation with Workers' Compensation. I suspected early on that my pharmacy would be a peripheral player. The real battle, I was sure, was going to be between the Christian God and the Imaging God.

I sent a note to the orthopedist opining that her pain was certainly the product of the fall and probably equally the product of her divorce. Whatever dynamic or combination of dynamics was involved, however, I certainly accepted her suffering. I did not believe she was a malingerer.

My therapy helped only a bit. There were too many other forces operative in her illness. She had faith that her God would cure her and also faith, I am sure, that He would allow her to receive a settlement from Workers' Compensation. This is the terrible fulcrum on which so much of the care of the painful rests. The effort to recover is balanced unfavorably by the effort to achieve other satisfactions. However, to identify patients who are seeking recompense for their injuries as malingerers just because we do not understand the nature of their illness is not only unscientific—it is unchristian.

> *To identify patients who are seeking recompense for their injuries as malingerers just because we do not understand the nature of their illness is not only unscientific— it is unchristian.*

Another player came on the scene, the Insurance God. I was not to be a provider under her state-sponsored indigent medical care plan. Other doctors would attend her. Their tests were negative, and their therapies ineffective. She kept in touch with me, writing occasional letters, describing her pain and her plight and requesting my support in her litigation. Her attorney asked that I provide an impairment rating, a statement quantifying her disability, this toward reaching a financial settlement with Workers' Compensation.

Disability evaluations are supposed to be scientific. There are tables and combinations of tables that allow, on the basis of imaging studies and clinical evaluation, an exact measure of impairment. The tables do afford physician discretion, however, and I was generous with Georgia. The aggregate effect of her injuries amounted, according to my calculations, to a 20 percent impairment. This is a very high disability rating, and the financial settlement, considering her resources, would be large.

My judgments, so favorable to Georgia, were the product of simple observational science. Her life had been wrecked by an injury. The validity of that observation was incontestable. The normal MRI was, in my judgment, irrelevant. Later, in deposition, I was taken to task for my generous impairment rating. The insurance company's attorneys pointed out that the physicians who had assumed her care after she left me had also provided ratings. Both of them, using the same tables that I did, derived an impairment rating of zero. Her imaging studies were normal, and she was, therefore, not impaired.

We don't give the painful, particularly the unaccountably painful, the respect they deserve. We continue to demand that they demonstrate that their suffering is due to something we can understand. In the absence of pathologic accountability for pain, we treat the patient with suspicion. Painful patients are the object of rejection, distrust, and injustice. This is the reason they so often just give up.

Molly suffered continued pain following surgery for a herniated lumbar disc. Our interview was laborious—the woman had a wall around her. Her mind-soul was not to be easily penetrated. She was a nurse and knowledgeable in matters of the body. She could not understand why removal of the disc had not cured her pain. Her post-operative imaging studies were normal, but there had to be some pressure on a nerve to make her hurt this way. She was agreeable to my interview, but there was no embrace. She was taciturn, frank, and it seemed void of any emotional force. I extracted her history very slowly.

She was hearing-impaired from childhood mumps. Her parents were alcoholic and subject to erratic behaviors. As a teenager, Molly occasionally slept on the streets to get away. She graduated, with difficulty, from nursing school and found employment in a rural medical clinic. She acknowledged that she had suffered moodiness throughout her life and had always been sleep-deprived and appetite-irregular. Nonetheless, she was able to work rather effec-tively. Her painfulness was late onset, appearing about age forty. It occurred after her clinic downsized and her employment termi-nated. With that event came depression, and an unsuccessful operation.

"My doctors can't find what is wrong with me. The surgery only made me worse. There has to be something wrong in there, but they can't find it. Can you find it? I know it is there. I am a nurse. I know these things. You don't feel the pain I feel unless something is wrong in there."

She was a tough interview. She never opened up. She had distrust and suspicion written all over her. I went slowly, but I did ask if she had ever suffered sexual abuse during her childhood. She acknowledged, without any display of emotion, that there was an event that bothered her. Each summer she went to visit her grand-father. These were pleasant stays, but on one occasion he had friends over to play cards. She remembered the beer cans, the poker chips, and the laughing, loud old men. They included her in the game and dealt her some cards. She won the pot. Then Grandfather turned on the phonograph and lifted six-year-old Molly onto the table to dance for his friends. She remembered their applause. Grandfather took her upstairs to bed. She couldn't remember exactly what happened after that.

I didn't dwell with her on that event nor did I suggest it had any relevance to her painfulness. That would have been destructive. No need to suggest that her pain was the product of a tortured mind when she knew quite well that it was due to a tortured nerve in her back. We concluded a long interview, and I told her there were prospects for improvement. Molly was a redoubtable woman. She had achieved much in a handicapped life. The infrastructure was intact. If strength of character is a measure of recovery, Molly certainly had that. I was rising to the challenge as a fish rises to the bait.

She called the next day to cancel her return appointment. This happens a lot. Since we are into statistics, probably about 20 percent of the time. Painful patients give up easily. Distrustful and suspicious already, they become more so when I conduct my interview. "Dr. Jones told me you could help me with my pinched nerves. Why are you asking me these questions? Are you some kind of psychiatrist?"

The physician, encountering a patient with recurrent chest pains, begins his analysis with pointed interrogation. The location, character, and the inciting events which precipitate pain are recorded. Suspecting coronary artery disease, he will question regarding the antecedents of tobacco use or a family history of coronary disease. He will inquire as to the comorbidities of diabetes and hypertension. These interrogations are appropriate and warranted. To omit them would be dereliction.

The physician, encountering a patient with chronic pain, asks of its location, character, and duration. He should also make inquiries into the existence of risk factors such as depression, drug dependency, and childhood abuse. These antecedents bear the same relationship to the generation of chronic pain as the antecedents of tobacco, hypertension, diabetes, and high cholesterol do in the generation of coronary disease. To omit their investigation is dereliction.

Such interrogations often represent, in the mind of the patient, a threat and an intrusion. The search for the origin of pain in the mind rather than the body can be a humiliating experience to endure. Nonetheless, most patients cooperate with the inquiry. They recognize it as a new and hopeful avenue of discovery. In a few, however, the threat is too great. It was in Molly. She never accused me of being a psychiatrist. She was so incapable of emotional display that she never addressed the issue. She just gave up.

I am wrong a lot, but occasionally I am right, and I was right about Molly. Strength of character is important. Molly had decided that maybe she had made a mistake, that maybe there was something to this drug business. She showed up a couple of months later. Her behaviors were as before, strict, controlled, and void of reaction. There was candor, but there was no warmth, nor was there ingratiation.

"I went ahead and took your medicine, and I did sleep better. I think it was helping my damaged nerve. When I used it all up, my pain got worse. Can you give me some more?"

I wrote her another prescription but told her that there would be no refills until she returned for follow-up. I was frank and to the point with Molly, just as she had been with me. I renewed her Imipramine and Klonopin and later added an opiate, Methadone. (Yes, there is a place for opiates. Opiates on top of mind-soul drugs can be very helpful. Mind-soul drugs on top of opiates, however, rarely work.) I assisted an attorney in obtaining her disability benefits, and Molly, retired from nursing, found a new endeavor—cake decorating. With each visit, as she entered a sort of recovery, she became more engaging and open, and more curious about her illness.

"My pain wasn't due to a damaged nerve, was it? It was due to something that happened in my mind, in my brain chemistry."

"Yes, Molly. That is correct."

"I want to tell you something."

"What is that?"

"You are the only doctor I have ever seen who thought I was worth caring for. Thank you for being so compassionate."

This kind of declaration, and I hear it a lot, is the mind-soul of the painful patient finding expression. The disease, its antecedents, and often its treatments inflict confusion, shame, indignity, and suspicion on its victims. No other illness is so destructive to the sense of self-worth.

"Thank you, Molly. Thank you very much. I appreciate your compliment, but you are wrong, Molly. Your physicians, all of them, are wonderful people. They did the best they could. They did not want for compassion, but I am afraid, Molly, that sometimes they want for understanding. It is their training. They were taught from the time they entered medical school, just as you were taught from the time you entered nursing school, that pain was always due to damaged tissue, and if the damage could be repaired by rest, injection, or by surgery, the pain would go away. They have been taught wrong, Molly. There is a lot more to pain than damaged tissue."

For the first time I saw her smile. "Yes, Dr. Bob, I can see that now."

Epilogue

The prescription of drugs for the treatment of disease always entails risk. Although the prospect for success may be high, the prospect for adverse reactions is never insignificant. This is particularly so in chronic pain, for it is the disease, above all others, which demands the greatest number and variety of drugs. Although I have written with enthusiasm about their utility, I have not ignored their side effects. Some, such as sedation and sexual dysfunction, are highly inconveniencing; others, such as addiction, mania, or sucidial ideation, are truly catastrophic. For this reason, *the reader with chronic pain is admonished to avoid the self-administration of drugs.* The prescription of pharmacy should be left in the hands of competent professionals.

As medical science has evolved away from the belief in a mind-body dichotomy, there has occurred a melding of psychiatric science with other medical disciplines. The internists, neurologists, and anesthesiologists who have traditionally managed the patient with chronic pain are becoming increasingly sophisticated in the use of mind-soul drugs. At the same time, psychiatrists, already skilled in the use of the drugs, are learning how to employ them for such nonpsychiatric disorders as fibromyalgia and reflex sympathetic dystrophy.

These are the new medical specialists, physicians dedicated to the study and treatment of chronic pain. There are increasingly more of them, and they are getting better and better at their craft. Seek them out and tell them your story—your whole story. Hold nothing back and be patient, for there is no quick or easy fix to chronic pain. You must persevere, and if you do, they will probably help you find an answer—there usually is one.

About the Author

A graduate of Vanderbilt University Medical School, Robert T. Cochran Jr., M.D., completed his residency in internal medicine and neurology at the University of Texas and Duke University. In 1963, he established his private medical practice in Nashville, where he continues to work today.

Serving as the co-director of the Pain Center at Centennial Hospital in Nashville in the 1990s, Dr. Cochran built a reputation as a leader in chronic pain treatment. Treating thousands of pain patients throughout his forty-year practice has enabled him to explore the commonality of all chronic pain sufferers, as well as understand the real scope of painfulness.

Dr. Cochran uniquely incorporates the fields of neurology, internal medicine, and psychiatry in deriving insightful—sometimes disturbing yet hopeful—conclusions for the chronic pain sufferer. He brings to light intriguing new treatment strategies that should be of interest to the medical community and chronic pain sufferers alike.

Dr. Cochran and his wife, Donna, reside in Nashville. They have three children and seven grandchildren.

For additional information, go to Dr. Cochran's Web site, www.understandingpain.com.